Infant Nutrition

Infant Nutrition

Edited by
ANN F. WALKER
Department of Food Science and Technology
The University of Reading, Reading, UK

and

BRIAN A. ROLLS
Institute of Food Research, Reading Laboratory
Reading, UK

A Chapman & Hall Food Science Book

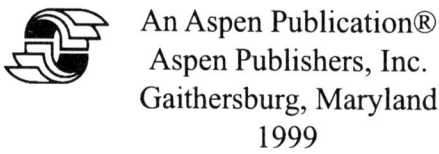
An Aspen Publication®
Aspen Publishers, Inc.
Gaithersburg, Maryland
1999

Originally published : New York : Chapman & Hall, 1994.
Includes bibliographical references and index.
(Formerly published by Chapman & Hall, ISBN 0-412-59140-5) ISBN 0-8342-1359-1

94-70922
CIP

About Aspen Publishers • For more than 35 years, Aspen has been a leading professional publisher in a variety of disciplines. Aspen's vast information resources are available in both print and electronic formats. We are committed to providing the highest quality information available in the most appropriate format for our customers. Visit Aspen's Internet site for more information resources, directories, articles, and a searchable version of Aspen's full catalog, including the most recent publications: **http://www.aspenpublishers.com**
Aspen Publishers, Inc. • The hallmark of quality in publishing
Member of the worldwide Wolters Kluwer group

Editorial Services: Ruth Bloom
Library of Congress Catalog Card Number: 94-70922
ISBN: 0-8342-1359-1
Printed in Great Britain at St Edmunsbury Press
1   2   3   4   5

Contents

Contributors

A. ASHWORTH

Centre for Human Nutrition, London School of Hygiene and Tropical Medicine, Keppel Street, London WC1E 7HT, UK

W.F.J. CUTHBERTSON

Harefield, Middlesex, UK

P.S.W. DAVIES

MRC Dunn Nutrition Centre, Downham's Lane, Milton Road, Cambridge CB4 1XJ, UK

A. DRAPER

World Cancer Research Fund, 11–12 Buckingham Gate, London SW1E 6LB, UK

S. FILTEAU

Centre for International Child Health, Institute of Child Health, 30 Guilford Street, London WC1N 1EH, UK

J. KING

Cancer Research Campaign, 10 Cambridge Terrace, London NW1 4JL, UK

D.A. MONERET-VAUTRIN

Service de Médecine 'D', Immunologie Clinique et Allergologie, Hôpital de Brabois, 54511 Vandoeuvre-les-Nancy, France

J.B. MORGAN

School of Biological Sciences, University of Surrey, Guildford GU2 5XH, UK

A.A. PAUL

MRC Dunn Nutrition Centre, Downham's Lane, Milton Road, Cambridge CB4 1XJ, UK

E.M.E. POSKITT

MRC Dunn Nutrition Unit, Keneba, Fajara, nr Banjul, PO Box 273, The Gambia

J. RIBY

College of Natural Resources, Agricultural Experimental Station, Department of Nutritional Sciences, University of California, Berkeley, CA 94720, USA

A. TOMKINS

Centre for International Child Health, Institute of Child Health, 30 Guilford Street, London WC1N 1EH, UK

R.G. WHITEHEAD

MRC Dunn Nutrition Centre, Downham's Lane, Milton Road, Cambridge CB4 1XJ, UK

Preface

Few people doubt that the mother's milk provides the best food for the full-term infant during the first few months of life, when the digestive, absorptive and excretory systems are relatively immature. The development of the digestive enzymes is detailed in Chapter 4. The significance of this immaturity first emerged as a consequence of the pioneering work of Professor Robert McCance and Dr Elsie Widdowson in human nutrition, when they studied the electrolyte and nitrogen excretion of babies and young animals. To quote Professor McCance, 'Inefficient though the kidneys were by adult standards, they were capable of maintaining homeostasis, **provided the infant and animals were growing while being fed on food of exactly the right composition – that is, the milk of the mother.**' (Ashwell, 1993).

One should not forget that although the mother protects the developing baby against much nutritional abuse, the baby may be still be affected by maternal nutrition, and this is discussed in Chapter 2.

The superior qualities of breast milk are still recognized, and research continues to discover yet more factors in breast milk significant to the health of the baby for possible inclusion in formulas. The immature stage of development of the baby means that while enough nutrients for optimal growth of all tissues are required, excessive quantities may cause intoxication. Tight specifications are essential, since unlike the adult the newborn depends on a single food. The slow and sometimes painful development of infant formulas is described in Chapter 1, and in Chapter 5 we are reminded that our knowledge of the nutrient requirements of infants is continuously being updated.

There is probably no other time in life when diet and health are so intimately related, a topic covered in Chapter 6. Human milk not only provides the 'model' for formulating infant foods for those who cannot, for whatever reason, be breast fed, but has other benefits to health that have so far escaped replication. Although cows' milk has provided the basis for infant feeds, there are important compositional differences from human milk, as Chapter 7 indicates.

As well as containing many factors to enhance immunity, it is widely believed that breast-fed infants are protected against allergic response, which seems to be an increasing problem in Western societies. Cows' milk contains more than twenty proteins, of which five may be allergenic, but substitutes such as goats' milk or soya products may also provoke response. Chapter 8 explores the problems of allergic response in infants.

Chapter 3 reminds us of the considerable variation in infant feeding practices in the world. In many Third World countries, it may not be possible to prepare infant formulas hygienically, and breast feeding assumes an even greater importance. For any infant, weaning is an important stage, depending much on the infant's physiological and psychosocial development. However, in the Third World the infant may be challenged with infant foods of low energy density and poor hygiene, leading to malnutrition (see Chapter 9). In the developing world, breast-fed infants are largely protected against diarrhoea, but it is so common at weaning that it has become known as the 'weaning disease'. The provision of safe, nutritious weaning food needs urgent attention and sound local solutions.

We hope that this book will provide an insight into the problems and some of the solutions associated with infant feeding in both Western and developing worlds.

Ann Walker
Brian Rolls

Ashwell, M. (1993) *McCance and Widdowson: A Scientific Partnership of 60 Years*. London, British Nutrition Foundation.

1
Infant foods in the United Kingdom from Victorian times to the present day

W.F.J. Cuthbertson
Harefield, Middlesex, UK

INTRODUCTION

This chapter summarizes changes that occurred during the last century in feeding normal full-term infants, i.e. those not afflicted with prematurity or metabolic, immunological or other handicaps.

Infant feeding is a far from simple operation in that the methods or foods used must conform with a variety of criteria which change as the infant develops and may themselves be modified as fashions dictate and as knowledge of nutrition may suggest. Whatever the circumstances several major conditions must be met. Moreover, these constraints must be met whether the infant is at the breast or artificially reared, and whether given home-made or commercial foods.

1. The food will not be given if any adverse effects are suspected or if it is not acceptable to the infant: no food has any nutritional value until it is consumed!
2. It must be available in the amounts required and at costs, in time or money, affordable.
3. It must be satisfactory in its method of preparation and consistent in its quality (appearance, odour and even taste) as judged by the carers, whether the mother, other family members or paid helpers.
4. It must conform, so far as possible, with advice given to the carers whether from experienced grandmothers or neighbours, statements in

Infant Nutrition. Edited by A.F. Walker and B.A. Rolls.
Published in 1994 by Chapman & Hall, London.
ISBN 0 412 59140 5.

the media or professional sources such as the mother and child welfare centres.

Infant feeding procedures might thus be expected to change but slowly. However, during the last 100 years there have been considerable modifications and some of them have occurred within a very few years of first recommendation. During this period there has been a more than tenfold reduction in infant mortality. Many factors have been involved. Of these, infant nutrition, although of major importance, is only one.

Between 1838, when records began, and 1900 infant mortality in England and Wales was static, at about 140–160 per 1000 live births in the first 12 months, i.e. that of a developing country of the present time. Although most babies were then breast-fed some, for a variety of reasons, were not.

Infant foods were then of low quality because of ignorance of infant nutrition and the varying composition and dubious origins of the major infant food ingredient, cows' milk, which was unpasteurized, microbially contaminated and often diluted and adulterated. The mortality of hand-fed babies was very high: 200–300 per 1000. In fact, it is remarkable that as many as 70–80% survived the nutritional insults and microbial challenges to which they were subjected.

From the turn of the century there has been a continuing decrease in mortality in the UK, where it is now about eight per 1000 (Central Statistical Office, 1990). It is not possible to attribute this improvement to any one factor. Most of the mortality resulted from infections of many types, although gastrointestinal disorders were dominant.

Although the production and use of improved infant foods have been of great benefit, the control of infant diseases has been brought about by a variety of means. These measures were introduced progressively, some as a direct consequence of legal enactments or public health measures, while others resulted from improvements associated with increases in the standard of living during this period. Some of these are as follows:

Improvements in milk quality
1. Introduction of methods for chemical and microbial
   evaluation   1900s
2. Introduction of pasteurization   1900s
3. Cold storage of bulk milk   1900s
4. Sale of pasteurized milk in sealed bottles   1930s
5. Control of bovine tuberculosis and brucellosis   1930s

Improvements in infant foods
1. Roller-dried pathogen-free milk to be made up
   with pathogen-free (70 °C) water   1900s

2. Use of nutrient supplements (fruit juices and
   cod liver oil)   1900s
3. Addition of vitamin D and iron to the foods   1920s
4. Use of low-electrolyte formulations   1970s

Control of transmission of infections
1. Microbially safe water supplies   1900s
2. Safe disposal of sewage   1900s
3. Decrease of flies by replacement of horse-drawn
   by mechanical transport   1930s

General health measures
1. Vaccination of infants   1930s
2. Reduction of numbers of infected individuals
   in the general population   1900s
3. Use of antibiotic treatments   1930s
4. Use of refrigeration in the household   1950s
5. Last, but not least, female literacy and
   increasing awareness, until recently, of the dangers   From
   of microorganisms, the importance of cleanliness and   early
   fresh air encouraged by all the media   1900s

THE HISTORY OF INFANT FEEDING IN THE UNITED KINGDOM FROM VICTORIAN TIMES TO THE PRESENT DAY

Breast feeding

The value of breast milk for the normal full-term infant depends on its nutritional and anti-infective properties.

Although lactational ability may vary greatly from mother to mother, almost all are able to provide ample milk for the first 6 months or so, after which the infant's needs often outpace the mother's ability to lactate. Then, although breast feeding is normally desirable to ensure optimal progress through the weaning period, additional food may become essential.

The anti-infective properties of breast milk are often as important as its nutritional attributes. During pregnancy, immunoglobulin G (IgG) is transferred across the placental membranes, conferring passive immunity against those systemic diseases to which the mother had been exposed. Gastrointestinal infections in the mother induce proliferation of lymphoblasts able to produce immune bodies. These cells then enter the systemic circulation to lodge in a variety of mucosal tissues (gut, lactating mammary gland, lungs, uterine cervix and lachrymal glands), where they produce secretory immunoglobulin A (sIgA), the major component of colostrum and of the whey protein moiety of mature breast milk. This sIgA is not degraded in the infant alimentary tract and so protects the children from all those gastrointestinal and upper respiratory tract infections to which the mother had successfully responded (Kenny *et al.* 1967; Ogra *et al.* 1977; McClelland *et al.* 1978; Hanson *et al.* 1982).

In subsistence and developing economies (whether at present in the developing world, or in Victorian times in the UK), by far the greatest investment is in children. This is not only for the pleasure which they provide but also because a family may offer the only safeguard for the parents against penury and starvation or the shame of a pauper's existence in ill health or old age. Apart from this, in such environments children soon contribute to family life by fetching wood or water, tending stock in the field or even as child labour, contributing to the family income from the age of 7 or even 5.

Under such circumstances breast feeding is the norm. A small proportion of mothers may be physiologically unable to lactate, while others may not breast feed because of disease or economic reasons such as the need to undertake work incompatible with breast feeding in order to earn enough to support other family members. For such mothers, and for the wealthy not wishing to breast feed, a wet-nurse was commonly the best choice for the child, but in her absence a breast milk substitute would be essential to save the baby's life. In such emergencies the milk of various animals such as the cow, and farinaceous foods and paps made with milk or water were commonly employed (Drummond and Wilbraham, 1939; Fildes, 1986). However, such home-made preparations, like those now made in some developing countries, are so much trouble to make that it is hard to believe that any mother would use them if she could breast feed in the normal way. Another method, probably employed more often to supplement the breast, or to assist weaning, was the use of mouth-to-mouth transfer of pre-chewed food from the mother (or nurse) to the infant (Drummond and Wilbraham, 1939; Fildes, 1986). It is tempting to speculate that this custom may have been vitally important in the hunter–gatherer phase of man's evolution and that the modern pleasure in kissing may be an atavistic remnant of this primordial necessity!

Victorian England: a developing country

During the 19th century cereal preparations with skim or full cream milk and added water or barley water were commonly used in the UK. Dried, cooked and malted cereal preparations began to be manufactured in 1860–1870 and were offered as 'patent' or 'proprietary' foods to be mixed with milk or water and used for infant feeding. In the 1870s 'tinned' sweetened condensed milk became available because of developments in its manufacture from skim milk, which was a by-product from butter factories. Its preservation was achieved by addition of sucrose in hermetically sealed tinned steel cans ('tins' in the UK, 'cans' in the USA). Developments in canning technology then permitted production at the rate of 1000 tins per person per day as compared with a rate of only 60 per person per day in the 1840s (Cuthbertson, 1982).

These technical advances encouraged the use of products much simpler to prepare and use than the paps and milk recipes previously employed, but similar grave disadvantages were to follow their use.

Cheadle (1889) and Barlow (1894) clearly differentiated rickets from scurvy and noted the association between the use of farinaceous and skim milk foods with the prevalence of these infant afflictions. Barlow (1894) attributed the increase in scurvy noted after 1870 (especially in the better-off families) to the use of preserved 'proprietary' foods by the well-to-do as compared with the poor, who were forced to use potato in their paps rather than the expensive proprietary foods. Barlow (1894) reported the rapid resolution of infant scurvy by fresh foods such as milk and meat juices, although he noted these were not as efficacious as vegetable and fruit juices.

Rickets was common in the 19th century even amongst the breast-fed because of dietary vitamin D deficiency and lack of exposure to sunshine in mothers. Cod liver oils were first used for 'rheumatism', i.e. pains in the joints, some of which may have been caused by rickets or osteomalacia. The remedy was not at first widely used, as the earlier products were obtained from rotted livers and were dark, revolting fluids. Fox, in 1848, discovered that a paler and less objectionable oil could be made from steamed, fresh livers and so encouraged wider use of this agent. Cheadle (1889) demonstrated that these preparations cured rickets in infants, while in 1889 Bland Sutton (quoted by Cheadle, 1902), showed it to be equally effective in the treatment of rickets in lion cubs at the London Zoo!

Dried full cream milk powder was first made by Grimwade in 1847 (Barber and Page, 1982). Vacuum concentration of milk at low temperature (71 °C, 160 °F) formed a dough-like mass which, when cool, set to a solid that could be ground to a powder. Although commercially available from the 1860s it was largely replaced in the 1870s by canned condensed milk made by the Borden process. The Grimwade type method was, however, employed in the production of at least one type of malted milk food from the 1890s to the 1950s (Anon. 1898, 1953).

It was not until the start of the 20th century (1902) that Just and Hatmaker devised the roller drying process for the cheap and effective production of full-fat dried milk products which proved to be the major basis for artificial infant foods during the first seven decades of the 20th century (Drummond and Wilbraham, 1939; Jephcott, 1969).

Towards the end of the 19th century, calorimetric investigations, notably those of Atwater and Voit (Hutchinson, 1900–1906) had determined to a high degree of precision the energy value of many foods and of their component fats, proteins, starches and sugars. These data were successfully applied to the prediction of food needs for adults. However, there was no clear understanding that for infants starch differs from the simple sugars in that it is not digested by the very young even after cooking (Coutts and Baker, 1914). This is in spite of the fact that since 1878 many of the authorities quoted by Coutts and Baker (1914) had shown that diets rich in starch and low in fat were most unsatisfactory.

Pasteur in the 1860s had shown that heat treatment at 70 °C destroyed vegetative organisms and so could prevent deterioration of wine. Later this process of pasteurization was shown to destroy milk-souring organisms and so the method was employed by the larger dairy companies in Europe and the USA to prolong the life of this highly perishable commodity. These same dairy companies realized in the 1890s that pasteurization could have a public health benefit in that it destroyed pathogens as well as the souring organisms (Drummond and Wilbraham, 1939).

As a result the process was encouraged by the public health authorities although there was a great deal of resistance to this procedure (Wilson, 1942), on much the same grounds as the criticisms now being levelled against radiation treatment for preservation or extending shelf life.

Milk was frequently adulterated, usually by removal of fat and addition of water together with preservatives such as formaldehyde, borax and salicylates (Willoughby, 1903; Tibbles, 1907; Dingwall-Fordyce, 1908).

The germ theory of disease had a great influence on life towards the end of the 19th century. This led not only to more attention to cleanliness and hygiene but also to the use of heat treatment for infant foods, often resulting in the use of 'preserved' foods characterized by destruction of antiscorbutic action or loss of 'freshness' (Barlow, 1894; Cheadle, 1889; Cautley, 1896, 1903).

Although the importance of nutrition was being recognized at this time, there were many unsolved problems. Scurvy was generally agreed to result from a shortage of something associated with 'fresh' foods, but there was a dispute over rickets. Some thought it to be caused by a shortage of fat: was it not cured by cream and cod liver oil? Others believed it to be a microbial infection: was it not prevented and cured by fresh air and exercise? Starch presented other difficulties. Precise work with humans and animals had clearly proved its value for them, so how could it possibly be without benefit for the infant?

In the 1860s Liebig had shown, by work with animals and people, that food owed its value to its carbonaceous, nitrogenous and mineral components. He then devised a 'perfect' infant food based on his analysis of breast milk: a mix of wheat and malt flour together with milk and potassium bicarbonate. When this was found not to be satisfactory in practice it was protested that this failure could not be supported on theoretical grounds because 'the new food contains the very same ingredients as mothers' milk and since this food agrees with them I cannot understand why they should be unable to digest Liebig's food' (Drummond and Wilbraham, 1939).

One cannot help feeling that because the work on the use of starch by adults was so obviously true many thought that starch *must* be utilized by infants, even though clinical experience repeatedly showed otherwise. This is only one of many instances in which good laboratory and epidemiological observations have led to ineffective or harmful results when attempts were made to apply laboratory findings without properly conducted trials on the target populations. Many recommendations on dietary modifications resulting from general agreement or consensus (on the use of vitamins, protein, starch, fat, salt and sugar, for instance) have been changed or withdrawn as a result of large-scale applications of attractive but erroneous and inadequately tested theoretical arguments.

At the turn of the century therapeutic investigations depended on either epidemiological observations (e.g. Howarth, 1905) or clinical studies on individual patients (e.g. Barlow, 1894). Clinical trials involving comparisons between the progress of comparable groups of patients allocated to different treatments were still several decades in the future. It is difficult to understand why comparative trials, such as those used by Lind in the 18th century, were not more often employed. One may speculate that, for ethical reasons, the physician could only apply that treatment thought to be the best, thereby discouraging simultaneous application of different therapies to comparable patients. With hindsight, it is clear that many disputed problems could have been readily resolved by comparative trials.

Infant mortality

A major epidemiological study (Howarth, 1905) reported the conditions of life and causes of infant mortality during the period 1900–1903 in Derby, a typical prosperous English industrial town with 'extremely limited slums' and 'almost non-existent overcrowding' but with a 'large number of privies and pail closets, the objectionable odours of which are lessened, to some extent, by the large open space at the rear of all buildings'. At this time there was no running hot water and few bathrooms or internal water toilets, while kitchen facilities were extremely limited and domestic refrigerators non-existent. Insects such as flies and bluebottles would have been difficult or impossible to control in summer, while vermin such as rats, mice, fleas and lice would not have been uncommon.

Between November 1900 and November 1903 each of the 9189 births registered was recorded with, when possible, the type of sustenance given up to the age of 12 months. Infant mortality and cause of death were also noted. Of the 8343 children investigated, 5278 were entirely breast-fed for the whole 12 months, 1439 were provided with some artificial food, and 1626 infants were entirely hand-fed. The infant mortality observed in these groups is shown in Table 1.1.

These data may be typical of the incidence of infant disease under what may have been the better circumstances in English towns during the 19th century. Breast feeding can be seen to lead to a considerable reduction in overall infant mortality. In the wholly breast-fed mortality was reduced to about a third, while even in the partly breast-fed the mortality was halved in comparison with the wholly artificially fed infants. Although especially marked for gastrointestinal and upper respiratory tract infections, the

Table 1.1 Effect of mode of nutrition on infant mortality in the UK, 1900–1903

	Breast-fed	*Hand-fed*	*Partly breast-fed, partly hand-fed*
Number	5278	1626	1439
Total mortality	368	321	142
Mortality	69.8	197.5	98.7

From Howarth (1905).
Of 9189 births there were 323 neonatal deaths, while the mode of nutrition of 523 living at 12 months, and of 17 infants dead at 12 months, could not be ascertained.

Table 1.2 Infant mortality amongst the 1626 hand-fed infants from Table 1.1

Diet	*Number*	*Deaths*	*Mortality*
Milk and water	895	158	177
All patent foods	422	85	202
Bread, rusks and other starchy food	159	40	252
Condensed milk	149	38	255
Incomplete data	1	0	0
Totals	1626	321	197.5

From Howarth (1905).
Mortality is expressed per thousand up to the age of 12 months.

benefits of breast feeding were also evident in all the disease groups recorded.

The foods provided for the hand-fed infants were noted and these observations are summarized in Table 1.2. Howarth (1905) remarks on the inadequacy of the starch-based foods whether proprietary or home-made and the poor performance on the sweetened condensed milk preparations whether skim or full cream because 'their low fat content results in slow starvation'. In these tests the 'fresh', household milk and water regimen offered the lowest mortality although this 'is not satisfactory' compared with breast feeding. He attributed the mortality and high levels of gastrointestinal disease in the milk-fed group to poor hygienic quality of the milk available and suggested that steps be taken to teach mothers the importance of hygiene.

Modification of 'fresh' cows' milk in the home would not have been easy at that time because of the great variation in fat (2–8%) and total solids (7–10.5%) of retailed milk (Willoughby, 1903; Dingwall-Fordyce, 1908). Moreover, in hot weather milk would often be 'on the turn', i.e. of high acidity from bacterial contamination so that 'scalding' to eliminate pathogens would induce coagulation of casein, thus making the milk impossible to feed through a teat from the bottle.

The decline of infant mortality after 1900

The standardized death rate from all causes at all ages between 1840 and 1870 remained at about 21 per 1000 live persons in England and Wales. After 1870 this mortality decreased, reaching about 17 per 1000 live persons by 1900 (Fig. 1.1). However, during this period the infant mortality (deaths per 1000 live births during the first 12 months) remained at 140–160 per 1000 with no perceptible trend between 1870 and 1900 (Fig. 1.2). After 1900 (Fig. 1.2), the infant mortality for England and Wales began to fall (Registrar General, 1908, 1911), and this decline has continued. In 1988 the infant mortality for England and Wales was only about one-fifteenth of the level observed in 1900–1902 (Table 1.3).

One can only speculate as to why this decline in infant mortality should have begun in 1900 but it was probably brought about by several simultaneous changes. During the last decade of the 19th century the importance of breast feeding was well recognized by almost all concerned with child welfare (Cheadle, 1889; Barlow, 1894; Cautley, 1896; Hutchison, 1900; Howarth, 1905), but since about 80% of mothers were already breast feeding there would appear to have been small room for improvement of this aspect of infant management (Barlow, 1894; Howarth, 1905; Dingwall-Fordyce, 1908).

The newer knowledge of nutrition, of the need for fat, protein, salts and

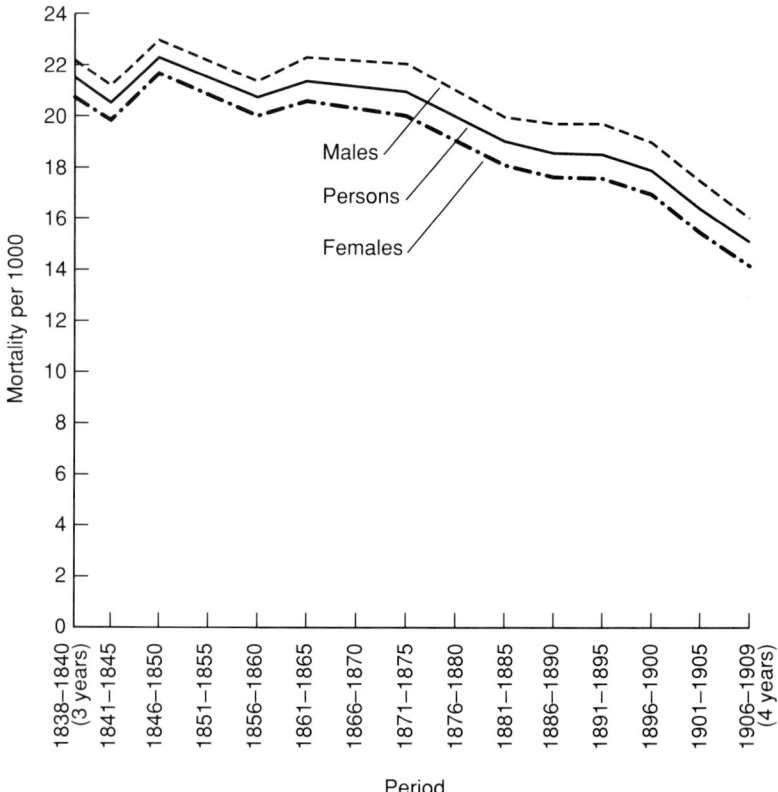

Figure 1.1 Corrected mortality in England and Wales between 1838 and 1909, plotted in 5-year periods. The death rates throughout the entire period are based on the age and sex constitution of the population in 1901. (From Registrar General, 1911.)

carbohydrate together with analyses then becoming available for human and cows' milk, led to the development of numerous recipes for breast milk substitutes to be made from cows' milk with the addition of water, fat and sugar (Cautley, 1903; Willoughby, 1903; Howarth, 1905; Dingwall-Fordyce, 1908; Coutts and Baker, 1914).

By the end of the 19th century the 'germ' theory of disease was well established in the public mind. At this time mains water and flush toilets were being installed. The harmful effects of cesspools, inadequate water supplies and flies as carriers of disease became recognized as well as the poor quality of the milk supply, which was then frequently infected with bovine tuberculosis and numerous other pathogens in addition to being adulterated with water and preservatives such as formaldehyde, borax and

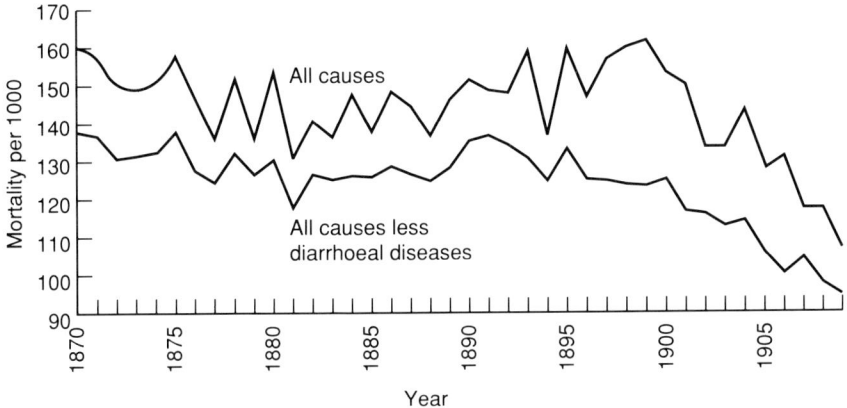

Figure 1.2 Infant mortality in England and Wales between 1870 and 1909, from all causes, and from all causes other than diarrhoeal diseases.(From Registrar General, 1911.)

salicylic acid (Willoughby, 1903; Tibbles, 1907).

The dangers of adulterated foods were publicly acknowledged while means of detecting adulteration, dilution and microbial contamination of foods in general and milk in particular were being developed. There were investigations sponsored by government to evaluate the problems, and legal measures were enacted to control harmful practices (Willoughby, 1903; Wilson, 1942).

Equipment for the major operations of the dairy industry

Table 1.3 Infant mortality in the UK, 1891–1988

Year	Mortality	Year	Mortality
1891–2	148	1910–12	110
1893–4	148	1920–2	82
1895–6	155	1930–2	67
1897–8	158	1940–2	59
1899–1900	158	1950–2	30
1901–2	142	1960–2	22
1903–4	138	1970–2	18
1905–6	130	1980–2	12
1907–8	119	1983–4	9.8
1909–10	109	1985–6	9.5
		1987–8	9.0

From Registrar General (1909) and Central Statistical Office (1990).
Mortality is express per thousand up to the age of 12 months.

became available in the closing years of the 19th century. Machines for fat separation, butter production, pasteurization, sterilization, heat exchange, refrigeration (without CFCs) and dispensing in sealed glass containers were all being introduced on a commercial scale (Willoughby, 1903). These appliances, together with standardization of procedures, improved transport and handling facilities, permitted increasing supplies of clean wholesome milk, although much of low quality continued to be retailed. Various special products, notably pasteurized and 'sterilized' milk in sealed bottles, as well as 'humanized' formulations designed for infant feeding, were on sale at the larger dairies in the major towns.

The inadequacy of artificial foods, especially the farinaceous proprietary types and the condensed milks, for infant feeding was well known (Cheadle, 1889; Barlow, 1894; Howarth, 1905). Although the infant mortality on milk foods was worse than at the breast, dried milk preparations could offer advantages in that the microbial hazards were decreased and mortality was far lower than on the starchy and farinaceous products (Howarth, 1905; Naish, 1908; Sheill, 1912).

A dried infant milk – a mixture of dried milk from which some of the casein had been removed and malt sugars added without starch – had been in use from 1893 (Dodd, 1892; Anon. 1893).

The baby-feeding bottles available in the 19th century were made of metal, glass, china or pottery to a wide variety of designs which were all difficult to clean, thus greatly hindering the administration of microbially tolerable liquid foods. It was not until 1898 that the easy-to-clean boat-shaped 'Allenbury' feeding bottle equipped with a sterilizable rubber teat and valve became available and thereby immensely simplified the task of feeding an infant hygienically on artificial milks (Fig. 1.3; Anon. 1898).

(This design remained dominant until about 1950, when it was displaced by the wide-necked bottles (Fig. 1.4) still used in 1990 and made of either glass or plastic. It is not known what induced this change – whether availability of wide bottles and teats, detergents to simplify cleaning, the dictates of fashion or a combination of these factors.)

Books on the newer knowledge of nutrition began to be published in the 1890s to disseminate information on nutrition and hygiene, often with special reference to the baby's particular problems. These publications were at first addressed mainly to the medical professions. There were many reprints and numerous revised editions were issued over the next two decades, together with others addressed to the lay person (Anon. 1908).

Public radio broadcasts (the 'wireless') would not be available until the 1920s and television not until the 1950s, but since the population of the UK was literate, newspapers, periodicals and women's magazines had

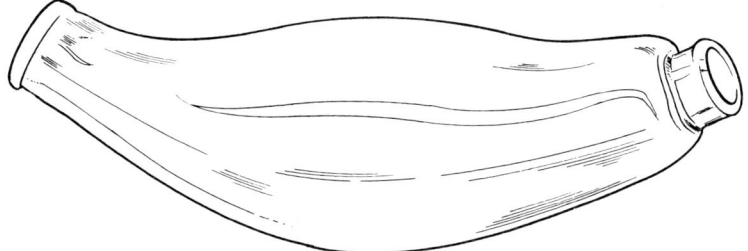

Figure 1.3 The Allenbury feeder, 1898. (From the Cow & Gate collection of feeding bottles. By permission, Cow & Gate Nutricia Ltd.)

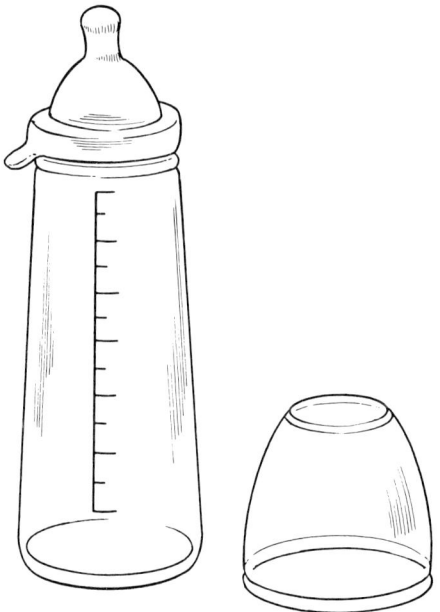

Figure 1.4 The Hygeia feeding bottle, with rubber teat and measuring lid, from the USA. (From the Cow & Gate collection of feeding bottles. By permission, Cow & Gate Nutricia Ltd.)

wide circulations and did much to extol the virtues of cleanliness, good hygiene and fresh air as well as advising mothers on the needs of their infants.

Hence by the end of the 19th century many of the causes of infant mortality and the means to avoid them were being recognized, widely publicized and increasingly applied. These changes, and their general appreciation, were probably in the Registrar General's mind when he stated in his report for 1906 that 'since the close of the century the subject of the waste of infant life, formerly treated with apathy, has received close and increasing attention from all classes of the community, and to this awakening may fairly be ascribed some portion of the decline in the rate of infantile mortality that has taken place during the past few years' (Registrar General, 1908). In the report for 1909 the Registrar General showed that the big decline in infant mortality since 1900 could not be associated with favourable climatic conditions, so that 'It is impossible to avoid associating this decline with the simultaneous effort to reduce infantile mortality' (Registrar General, 1911).

At that time (1900–1910) there were still serious problems in providing milk-based infant foods in the home. Even unadulterated milk from a reliable source would be of varying composition because of cream separation during delivery (by ladle from a churn) or in the jug at home. Furthermore, in those days of kitchens without refrigerators the rapid souring and coagulation of household milk in the summer would prevent the preparation of a liquid bottle-feed.

Dried milk powders were to help overcome these difficulties.

Roller-dried full cream milk powders

In 1902 Just and Hatmaker obtained patents for the production of dried milk by a process in which a stream of liquid milk is fed into the 'nip' between two rotating steam-heated hollow steel rollers. The milk first boils in the nip and then adheres as a damp but rapidly drying film on the rollers from which it is removed, in the form of a continuous sheet, by a knife (Fig. 1.5). This sheet of dried milk can then be ground to a powder for subsequent packing and convenience in use. This roller-dried product had advantages for the producer in that it could be made in large quantities during the flush milk season (spring and summer) when milk is cheap and under appropriate conditions could be kept for 18 months without significant loss of quality. For the consumer the benefit would be a dried milk of uniform quality free from harmful microbial contaminants.

Although the Just and Hatmaker patent was only granted in 1902 the advantages were so apparent that licenses to manufacture were rapidly negotiated and factories were planned, built and in production in New Zealand, the UK and Australia by 1904 in spite of a patent dispute and, in one instance, a set-back caused by a stick of dynamite thrown into the factory boiler by a disgruntled employee (Jephcott, 1969).

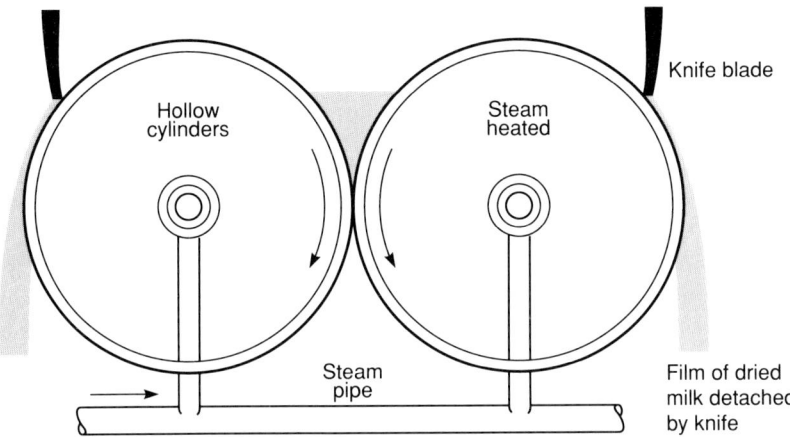

Figure 1.5 Principle of machine to produce roller-dried milk.

Sales of the milk powder failed dismally to meet expectations when it was offered as a replacement for liquid milk. However, trials of roller-dried milks in infant foods at the Finsbury Health Department were encouraging. As a result of these tests a modified formulation for use as an infant food was made by addition of lactose and cream to provide the required fat, protein and carbohydrate contents. This infant food (Glaxo) was sold only through pharmaceutical outlets (to ensure proper advice on its use), while a baby book (Anon. 1908) was printed and distributed to mothers as well as to nursing, medical and pharmaceutical professionals. In 1911 it was found that the use of a modified roller-dried full cream milk powder in place of cows' milk could lead to the elimination of the risk of 'summer diarrhoea', a dangerous infantile gastroenteritis commonly induced by infected milk in the summer months (Sheill, 1912). This roller-dried powdered infant food had several advantages over liquid milk (Naish, 1908; Sheill, 1912).

1. It was of a reliable, invariant composition.
2. It was simple to prepare: one measure per ounce of water.
3. Because of the heat treatment during manufacture the casein curd formed in the infant stomach was softer and less harmful than that formed from raw milk.
4. It could only be easily reconstituted in hot (>70 °C) water, so that no matter what the quality (or otherwise) of the local water supply the baby's food would be free from pathogens.
5. The food was sold through the pharmacy, so each purchase would offer an opportunity for advice.

6. The food was retailed in a reclosable tin, thereby preventing access of vermin or insects during storage in the home.
7. Instructions on use, and a measure, were provided in each tin and a book on baby care was available on request.

The first roller-dried infant foods did not fully meet the infant's needs in that they were marginally deficient in certain nutrients, notably ascorbic acid, vitamin D and iron. Some of the photographs published to show a healthy baby portrayed rachitic infants (Drummond and Wilbraham, 1939). However, the reduction in mortality that followed the assured supply of the major nutrients in a microbially safe food more than compensated for the occasional morbidity from these minor nutrient deficiencies. Within a few years supplements of fruit (or vegetable) juices, cod liver oil and iron were found to eliminate these problems of scurvy, rickets and anaemia.

Problems to be overcome in the manufacture and distribution of roller-dried milk products

The composition of cows' milk varies according to the season and the breed, stage of lactation and nutrition of the cow. Rapid methods of assaying the protein, fat and total solids content of the milk delivered from the supplying farms are therefore essential. Equipment to separate, or incorporate, the cream and sugar to produce a food of the calculated composition is also vital.

At the turn of the century reliable and rapid assays which could be carried out on numerous samples within the working day were available for nitrogen (total and precipitable), reducing sugars, ash, total solids and moisture. Equipment was available for precise temperature control (pasteurizers, heat exchangers, refrigerators), continuous cream separation, batch blending and prevention of cream separation during processing (Willoughby, 1903). The stage was thus set for the large-scale manufacture of milk products to precise analytical specifications. Further investigations were, however, essential before dried milk powders could be safely stored, distributed and used in the home.

The moisture content of milk powders is a major determinant of shelf life. At low moisture contents, oxidative rancidity is accelerated and leads to unpleasant rancid tastes and smells. At high moisture levels, Maillard reactions (between free amino groups of proteins and amino acids and reducing groups of carbohydrates) can lead to highly objectionable odours (of 'cardboard' and 'burnt feathers') as well as yellow and brown discoloration and loss of nutritional value.

Roller-dried full cream milk products containing 2.5–3.5% moisture can be stored at ambient temperatures of 10–20 °C for up to 18 months in the presence of air, without loss of quality. However, at lower or higher moisture contents there is serious risk of rapid loss of acceptability and nutritional value, and for these reasons a moisture-proof package is essential. Milk fat rapidly absorbs lipophilic odours, e.g. those of soap, engine oil, fruit, cheese and disinfectants. Thus, for safe transit, storage and display all packages (whether bulk or retail) must be impervious to objectionable odours, whether arising from other bulk items in a ship's hold or from scented or medicated goods on display in a retail pharmacy. For all these reasons milk powders could only be safely retailed in sealed impervious containers, i.e. tinned steel cans or glass jars, the former being much more common.

The specific volume, i.e. the volume occupied by unit weight of the product, needed precise control if the containers were to appear neither overfilled nor underfilled. More important was the fact that the mother, without precise scales, was advised to add a specified volume of powder (usually in a household measure such as a teaspoonful) to each volume of water (normally an ounce or tablespoonful) to give the required concentration of solids (often $\frac{1}{8}$ or $12\frac{1}{2}\%$) in the reconstituted infant food.

Roller-dried milk products are produced as voluminous sheets which are readily broken down to powder with a specific volume which can vary between wide limits depending on the degree and type of attrition employed. Thus, factory methods were needed that ensured the preparation of a powder which, even after further handling, transport, packaging, storage and use, would exhibit the specific volume essential if the measure used in the kitchen was to provide the weight of food needed. Recognizing the wide variation in kitchen equipment, some (but not all) manufacturers supplied a measure or gauge with each tin of baby food.

Packaging

Bulk packs

The packs and the materials of construction have changed over the years according to needs and availability (Warren, 1980). The first bulk packs were hessian or jute sacks lined with 'glassine' or grease-proof paper sacks, but these were unsatisfactory in not being proof against vermin (insects and rodents) or noxious vapours. The sacks were soon replaced by rectangular tinned steel boxes lined with grease-proofed paper and containing about 50 kg of powder. These tins were hermetically sealed with soldered or taped-on lids. During the 1930s the expensive tins were replaced by plywood kegs (tea chests) lined with paper and commonly containing about 25 kg.

After the Second World War 50 kg cylindrical fiberite drums lined with a sealed polythene (polyethene) bag were most often used. The fiberite provided protection against vermin and mechanical damage, while the heavy-duty polythene prevented ingress of moisture.

More recently multi-ply sacks have been increasingly employed. These generally consist of an inner, moisture-resistant barrier (often of poly-thene) and further layers, of waxed kraft paper (to prevent odour penetra-tion), plain kraft paper (to provide mechanical strength) and an outer kraft layer treated with a non-slip agent (to permit safe stacking). Though providing good protection from mechanical and chemical deterioration, these packs may be subject to insect or rodent depredations unless appro-priate precautions are taken. For instance, insect-proof heat sealing or stitching may be used for the sacks, or insecticides employed within the store.

Retail packs

Retail packs must protect the product as well as the bulk, while the quantity should be such that it will be used before exposure to ambient conditions can lead to any detectable deterioration (Warren, 1980). For these reasons baby foods are sold in small retail packs (150–1000 g), com-monly about 500 g), i.e. in sizes anticipated to last about a week. Packs should be reclosable, to offer protection from contamination and deterio-ration. Glass jars were at first employed for some of the smaller sizes (Anon. 1893), but the reclosable lever-lid tinned steel container (UK tins, US cans) was the almost universal pack from the beginning of the century (Anon. 1898, 1908). The baby food was weighed into a bag of sulphite 'parchment' or glassine paper to protect it from any traces of oil or solder left during fabrication of the tin. The bottom of the tin was then spun on hermetically to seal the container. The replaceable lever-lid was easily dis-placed to reveal the thin hermetic metal foil membrane that protected the contents and was scored to facilitate its removal and provide access to the food (Anon. 1906). Measures for the powder and for the water to dilute it were on sale (Anon. 1911), but spoons or measures for the solid powder were increasingly provided with the retail packs (Anon. 1908). Instructions for use were often printed on the pack, although a leaflet might be enclosed in the container. At first tins were covered by printed paper overwraps to protect them from rust and to illustrate and inform on use of the contents (Anon. 1898, 1908). By about 1920, enamelling tech-niques permitted direct printing on the metal to eliminate any need for a paper overwrap (Anon. 1920, 1925).

At a later date cans with slip-on lids sealed with adhesive tape came into common use; these did not provide a hermetic seal. Although the containers were not completely air-tight, the ingress of air and moisture was insufficient to affect the shelf life of the infant food.

As tin plate prices rose and the quality and availability of plastics changed, so tins were replaced by cartons. The infant milk powders were protected from moisture in a bag, usually of polythene or polypropylene within a board carton which itself was enveloped in a transparent over-wrap of cellophane to provide odour protection. By this time – the early 1960s – pest infestations in the home and in retail outlets were so uncommon that packs to protect against insect and rodent attack were no longer needed. This type of pack was thenceforward in use for almost all infant foods derived from full cream milk until their withdrawal from the UK market in the mid-1970s (Mettler, 1980a).

In the early 1970s ready-to-feed liquid preparations became available, at first only for hospital use but later on general sale. These preparations were presented in sterile form in glass jars with tamper-evident seals to provide sufficient milk for a single feed. The closure could be removed and replaced by a sterile teat fixture for feeding.

In the 1970s the traditional roller-dried infant foods based on full fat milk with added carbohydrate were replaced by other formulations to meet new beliefs relating to infant nutrition. These novel foods differed from the old in several respects, notably replacement of the butterfat by other oils containing considerably higher concentrations of polyunsaturated fatty acids. This change greatly increased the rate of development of oxidative rancidity in these foods, so that the required shelf life could no longer be achieved in an air pack but demanded packaging under inert gas in hermetically sealed containers.

Spray-dried infant milk foods

In 1872 Percy patented a process whereby a jet of milk is sprayed into a warm air current so that water evaporates to leave a fine suspension of milk solids which can be separated as spray-dried milk powder (Lovell, 1980). Although many improvements were made to the economics of this system, the spray-dried powders were not satisfactory in that they were difficult to disperse in water and the full cream milk powders were subject to rapid deterioration from oxidative rancidity when stored in air packs. During the Second World War, large amounts of spray-dried skim milk powder were made for the armed forces and for manufacturing, catering and domestic use. Consumption in the home dropped at the end of the war until Peeble, in 1954, patented the 'instant' process whereby, on exposure to moisture, the fine spray-dried powder particles are induced to agglomerate into large porous granules which are quickly wetted and easily dispersed in water. The development and application of the 'instant' process have been reviewed by Wulff (1980). Further detailed investigations of factors controlling the properties of spray-dried products permitted the manufacture of spray-dried full cream milk powders of good stability that were also dispersible in warm (40–45 °C) water rather than in the hot (>70 °C) water essential for reconstitution of the roller-dried powders (Mettler, 1980b). As a result of these developments, the roller-dried infant foods began to be replaced by spray-dried equivalents in the 1970s. This change was accelerated by the withdrawal from the market of the traditional roller-dried infant foods made by simple additions of fat and carbohydrate to full cream milk.

Development of modern infant formulas

The infant foods offered during the first half of this century were almost entirely derived from cows' milk by addition of fat and carbohydrate (lactose, sucrose or maltose) and diluted to resemble breast milk in its major components. Although many formulations were devised, few trials were published that compared the nutritive value of the various products.

The need for dietary supplements to improve nutritive status was recognized early in that fruit or vegetable juice supplements were almost invariably advised to avoid scurvy, and cod liver oil preparations to eliminate the risk of rickets. Vitamin D was added to infant foods in the mid-1920s, i.e. as soon as tests for vitamin D were developed and odourless preparations of this vitamin became available (Jephcott and Bacharach, 1926, 1928; Coward, 1985). Problems with iron-deficiency anaemia were recognized by the Medical Research Council (MacKay and Goodfellow, 1931). This difficulty was rapidly overcome by the addition of a ferric ammonium citrate to provide the necessary iron. Ascorbic acid was found not to be destroyed during roller drying but to be destabilized so that this vitamin rapidly disappeared from the product. However, it was found that if crystalline ascorbic acid were added to the dry infant milk powders it would be retained almost indefinitely (W.F.J. Cuthbertson, A.E. Mettler and G.A. Childs, unpublished results). The use of appropriate preparations and modes of addition could permit the production of infant milk powders with defined and stable concentrations of vitamin A (A.E. Mettler, G.A.Childs and W.F.J. Cuthbertson, unpublished results). These observations led to the addition of ascorbic acid and vitamin A to roller-dried infant foods in the 1960s and also offered an explanation of the early observations (Jephcott and Bacharach, 1921) that, under some circumstances, roller-dried full cream milk powder could prevent scurvy in guinea pigs.

The sales of roller-dried infant milk foods increased continuously from their first introduction in 1904. However, until the Second World War the commonest infant feeding regimen still depended on the use of diluted fresh milk to which sugar was added. During and after this war fresh milk was increasingly replaced by roller-dried full cream milk formulations until by the 1960s fresh milk was rarely used in foods for young babies (Whitehead and Paul, 1987). During this period many concerned with mother and child welfare came to believe there was little to choose between breast and bottle feeding and that the various brands of infant food (almost all based on roller-dried milk powder) scarcely differed except in price and appearance of the package.

Replacement of simple roller-dried infant milks

The first indication of unease occurred when Lightwood and Stapleton (1953) drew attention to the fact that even an essential nutrient, vitamin D, can be harmful. At that time, needlessly high concentrations of vitamin D were added to infant foods and supplements. The majority of infants thus received between 40 and 100 µg vitamin D per day without any apparent ill effect. However, in a small minority a serious affliction, idiopathic hypercalcaemia, was induced. This had all the characteristics of vitamin D toxicity, but with no evidence of any abnormal intake of the vitamin (Cuthbertson, 1963). The condition almost completely disappeared after 1957 when the vitamin D content of infant milk formulas was reduced to 1 µg/100 ml and of cereal weaning foods to about 15 µg/100 g.

Neonatal hypocalcaemia can lead to dangerous neonatal convulsions in the newborn and was found by Oppe and Redstone (1968) to be associated with the use of certain milk formulations. Barltrop and Oppe (1970) showed the condition to be related to the phosphate content of the infant food and it could be controlled either by a decrease in the phosphate or an increase in the calcium content.

Taitz and Byers (1972) drew attention to the high incidence in the UK of dangerous hypertonic dehydration in babies with gastroenteritis. They showed this to be caused by the use of over-concentrated feeds by the mother, coupled with needlessly high levels of protein and electrolytes (especially sodium) in the full cream milk powders popular at that time and known to be well tolerated by normal infants. Calculation of the effects of food and water intakes and insensible water losses on renal loads clearly indicated a very significant decrease in the risk from dehydration when low-electrolyte formulas were used, as well as an even greater safety to be secured by breast feeding (Shaw *et al.* 1973). These difficulties were exacerbated by the low, and falling, proportion of mothers breast feeding their babies (Whitehead and Paul, 1987).

It was probably these findings, as well as previous observations on idiopathic hypercalcaemia and neonatal hypocalcaemia, that led to the commissioning by the Department of Health and Social Security (DHSS) of a series of authoritative reports on topics concerned with infant nutrition (DHSS, 1974, 1977, 1980a, 1980b, 1981). These reviews outlined current practices in infant feeding up to 1974 and 1980 (DHSS, 1974, 1980b), and provided analyses of pooled samples of breast milk (DHSS, 1977) to extend and to check (by modern analytical methods) previously published work on breast milk components from other countries and the UK (Kon and Mawson, 1950; Macy *et al.* 1953). This was information essential to the assessment of infant nutrient requirements. These studies culminated in the publication (DHSS, 1980a) of nutritional guidelines for the composition of artificial milks intended for use by the infant as well as recommendations as to how novel formulations might be scrutinized without unnecessarily inhibiting or delaying the application of new findings for the manufacture of improved products.

Low-electrolyte infant formulas

Meanwhile infant food manufacturers responded so rapidly to the expressed need for low-electrolyte infant foods that by 1973–1974 little of the traditional infant food was sold, and none was available after 1977 when the government-subsidized milk of this type (National Dried Milk) was withdrawn from the market (DHSS, 1980b).

The first of the low-electrolyte modifications of traditional infant milks were produced simply by approximately halving the solids-not-fat (SNF) of the dried milk moiety of the food and replacing it with carbohydrate. This reduction in SNF led to reductions in several nutrients, e.g. water-soluble vitamins and trace elements as well as protein and electrolytes. These were then added to make up the shortfall to levels characteristic of the unmodified milk foods or, as recommendations were published, to the concentrations suggested by authoritative national or international bodies (e.g. Codex Alimentarius Commission, 1976; ESPGAN, 1977; DHSS, 1980a).

Demineralized whey formulas

The ratio of whey protein to casein is much higher in breast than in cows' milk. The essential amino acid contents of casein and whey proteins differ in that whey protein contains more cystine plus cysteine (DHSS, 1977). As a result the DHSS (1980a) report suggested that the whey protein content of infant foods should be increased so that the whey protein : casein ratio and the proportions of the essential amino acids in the total protein should more closely resemble the values characteristic of human milk. This recommendation is surprising in that a large proportion (15–20%) of the breast milk whey protein is in the form of sIgA, which has an immunological, protective function in the alimentary tract and is not degraded in the gut. Between 70% and 90% of the ingested sIgA can be recovered from the infant faeces, so its amino acid content can be of scant nutritional value (Kenny *et al.* 1967; Ogra *et al.* 1977; McClelland *et al.* 1978; Hanson *et al.* 1982). However, as a result of the DHSS (1980a) recommendations milk foods containing demineralized whey and whey protein concentrates were rapidly developed in the UK, but less so in other countries. Comprehensive comparative surveys of the nutritional characteristics of the infant formulas available in the UK during this period were published, and these also discussed the nutritional problems caused by the replacement of milk by demineralized whey proteins (Mettler, 1976, 1979, 1980a; Barr and Mettler, 1983).

Essential fatty acid requirements

Hansen *et al.* (1958) showed that essential fatty deficiency arises when linoleic acid provides less than 0.1% of the total energy content of the infant diet, and suggested that the requirement for linoleic acid should be 1% of the energy intake, even though symptoms were not discernible in infants receiving less.

Infant fatty acid deficiency has only been noted in one patient (a victim of kwashiorkor) apart from iatrogenic instances (DHSS, 1980a). This despite the fact that a majority of infants in North America, Northern Europe, Australia and New Zealand have for many years been reared on full cream and half cream milk preparations providing respectively about 1.6% or less of their energy from linoleic acid.

In linoleic acid deficiency, the ratio in cell membranes of eicosatrienoic acid to eicosatetraenoic (arachidonic) acid, i.e. the triene : tetraene ratio, is raised. A value of 0.4 has been arbitrarily defined as the upper limit of normality (Holman, 1972), although this can be further depressed as intake of linoleic acid is increased from 1% to 4%, 5% or more of dietary energy (Hansen *et al.* 1962). Fomon (1967) has remarked that this changing ratio may be merely a measure of dietary intake rather than physiological need. This arbitrary limit of 0.4 for the triene : tetraene ratio was not exceeded in a series of trials using infant foods containing no fat other than butterfat (DHSS, 1980a). As a result of these findings, the DHSS (1980a) recommended that 'the linoleic and α-linolenic acid content of any feed should provide at least 1% of the total energy of the food'.

Using substantially the same published information, other national and international authorities promulgated somewhat different recommendations. Table 1.4 shows the recommendations of the various authorities and the amounts of the essential fatty acids required in 100 ml of infant food prepared to meet the required specifications (Mettler, 1982).

Table 1.4 Recommended levels of fat and of essential fatty acids per 100 ml of infant food providing 293 kJ (70 kcal)

Authority	Codex (1976)	ESPGAN (1977)	IFA (1980)	DHSS (1980)
Total fat (g)				
minimum	2.3	2.7	2.3	2.3
maximum	4.2	4.1	4.2	5.0
Linoleic acid (mg)				
minimum	210	233	210	
maximum	–	–	–	1000
Linoleic plus linolenic acids (mg)				
minimum	–	–	–	78
maximum	–	–	–	
Linoleic acid (% of total energy)	2.7	3–6	3	–
Linoleic plus linolenic acids (% of total energy)	–	–	–	1

From Mettler (1982).

It is difficult to understand why the Codex Alimentarius Commission (1976), ESPGAN (1977) and IFA (1980) should have set essential fatty acid requirements so high. A major influence may have been the levels of essential fatty acids found in breast milk, mainly from North American and European mothers! ESPGAN (1977) states: 'Human milk in most parts of the world contains between 7% and 12% of total fat as linoleic acid (corresponding to 3–6% of total energy). This is the main reason why this level has been proposed as an advisable intake. It is recognized that reasons for regarding the concentration in human milk as optimal are not strong as the level is dependent on the mother's intake of polyunsaturated fat.'

Whether or not the recommendations of these authorities are justified, all infant foods now sold meet these guidelines because no infant food manufacturer could afford to offer for sale anything not meeting *all* recommendations.

It is regrettable that the high levels of essential fatty acids needed prevent the use of readily accessible milk (buffalo, cow, goat or sheep) from which otherwise satisfactory infant foods could be made in many areas using simple technology and locally available raw materials. Such foods would meet the needs of many in developing countries who are unable to purchase the excellent, but expensive, products common in the developed world.

Problems relating to manufacture and development of novel infant milk formulas

Formulation

In modern low-electrolyte infant milk formulas the cows' milk content is greatly reduced. As a result the quantity of many nutrients – B vitamins and trace elements for instance – previously supplied by the SNF component will also be diminished and, if need be, must be added to the formula to ensure that all are present in a sufficiency to satisfy the guidelines.

In all instances tests must ensure that these added nutrients do survive manufacturing processes and will be still present in the required amounts until the shelf life or 'use by' date, and that no harmful interactions have taken place between the added agent and other components of the formula, e.g. between trace elements and fats or vitamins. Problems have arisen from the varying stability of different forms of the vitamins, for instance folic acid, vitamin B_6 and vitamin A, and the finding that conditions for optimum stability of one vitamin may be unfavourable for another (W.F.J. Cuthbertson, A.E. Mettler and G.A. Childs, unpublished results).

Although the guidelines specify the amounts of certain trace elements that should be present in the food, nothing is said of the chemical form of these substances, even though it was well known that speciation could have major effects on bioavailability and toxicity. Apart from this, some trace elements, notably iron, copper and manganese, can encourage undesirable oxidative reactions leading to loss of several nutrients and development of oxidative rancidity. Indeed, the need for any addition of copper has been questioned (Cuthbertson, 1974) in view of the very large stores in the liver of the newborn (about 10 mg; Widdowson and Spray, 1951; Widdowson *et al.* 1972) and the rarity of copper deficiency. In fact, only one instance has been reported, and that in an infant with kwashiorkor (Wilson and Lahey, 1960; ESPGAN, 1977). Some of these and related difficulties have been considered by Cuthbertson (1974, 1978), Mettler (1982) and Barr and Mettler (1983).

It has been pointed out that although breast milk is quite properly taken to be the ideal food, it could not be officially commended for sale even if commercially available, because a large proportion of samples fail to meet guidelines. A majority of milks tested (DHSS, 1977) fail to meet 20 out of 27 components specified by the Codex Alimentarius Commission (1976), while few if any mother's milk samples would be anticipated to meet all the guidelines listed (Cuthbertson, 1978).

There are suggestions that infant well-being may require special nutrients not required by the adult, e.g. certain hormones, and carnitine and taurine (DHSS, 1980a; Mettler, 1982). Although no specific need for these substances is noted in any guidelines, at least one infant formula now contains added taurine even though no benefit has been shown to accrue from its presence.

Recent observations by Lucas *et al.* (1992) have shown that infants given breast milk had significantly greater intelligence quotients (IQ) at $7^1/_2$–8 years of age than those receiving none. This difference has been attributed to the need for exogenous supplies of metabolically essential members of the *n*–3 series of polyunsaturated fatty acids (PUFA) at periods of rapid brain growth. It has been shown that the concentration of the *n*–3 series is decreased in the cerebral cortex of formula-fed infants and that this difference may be caused not only by their lower content in present infant formulas but also by the high concentrations therein of the *n*–6 series of PUFA, which may inhibit synthesis of the required members of the *n*–3 series from the limited amounts of precursors available (Farquharson *et al.* 1992). These findings suggest there is still substance in the view attributed to Oliver Wendall Holmes that 'A pair of substantial mammary glands has the advantage over the two hemispheres of the most learned professor's brain in the art of compounding a nutritious fluid for infants.'

Packaging and presentation

Within the last 10 years the presentation of infant formulas has been greatly modified. Changes have occurred because of increased concentrations of polyunsaturated fatty acids, the availability of improved packaging materials, developments in packaging techniques (especially aseptic procedures) and the need better to meet the convenience of the user (baby and mother, father or nurse), as well as infant nutrition!

Developments in spray-drying technology permit production of milk and infant formulas in powder forms equally as resistant to atmospheric oxidation as their roller-dried predecessors. They have additional advantages for the mother in that they can be made up in lukewarm (30–40 °C) water and so dispense with the need to reconstitute at the high temperature (>70 °C) essential when roller-dried products are employed.

In the presence of air, the shelf lives of modern infant milk formulas are much shorter than those of their traditional counterparts. This is because the higher concentration of essential fatty acids in present formulas renders them more susceptible to oxidative rancidity, which is also encouraged by the addition of iron, copper and manganese now mandatory if present guidelines are to be met. These effects are exacerbated by restrictions on the use in infant foods of antioxidants and chelating agents permitted for prevention of oxidative rancidity in other foods. As a consequence, infant foods meeting the guidelines required package in inert gas, and so were at first presented in hermetically sealed wallets constructed from metal foil–plastic laminates or alternatively in hermetically sealed cans of the lever-lid type. All packs were under inert gas and often at reduced pressure. More recently, these packs have been almost completely replaced by ring-pull easy-opening cans of metal or laminate with a plastic lid to protect the contents of the opened can.

Whatever the type of container all, since about 1985, are 'tamper-evident', i.e. fabricated so that once opened the package cannot be resealed. These precautions safeguard against malicious interference on supermarket shelves.

For export markets and for emergency supplies longer shelf lives are mandatory. Products for these purposes may be stored in cans under reduced pressure, to prevent 'blowing' of the pack during air transport or storage at high altitudes. Alternatively the formula may be placed, *in vacuo* or under reduced inert gas pressure, in a heat-sealed wallet made of a multi-ply laminate of plastic and aluminium foils to prevent ingress of moisture, oxygen and odours. These wallets are themselves placed in a plastic or card container to protect from mechanical damage and provide tamper-evident protection.

Ready-to-feed products

In the late 1970s and early 1980s ready-to-feed (RTF) liquid preparations of infant formula became available, not for general sale, but to save labour and simplify work in the hospital 'kitchens' (Barr and Mettler, 1983). There were severe technical problems to be overcome in their preparation, in that they were required to conform strictly with the guidelines, to be sterile and to be easy to use with no additions or manipulations.

Tight controls over use of food additives, such as emulsifiers and thickening and suspending agents, presented considerable problems. Additional problems are caused by a severe heat treatment for a period long enough to provide a 12 log cycle reduction in spore count of *Clostridium botulinum*, i.e. enough to render the probability of an infected 100 ml vial to be reduced to one in 10 thousand million, even if the initial count was as high as 100 *C. botulinum* spores per 100 ml.

Even after proper heat treatment there is always a possibility of breakdown of sterility through imperfections in the wall or seals of the container. For such reasons the first RTF products were dispensed in glass jars so that any change in the contents would be immediately detectable. The cap was so constructed that any change in internal pressure, indicating microbial contamination, would also be quickly discernible. With increasing experience, however, preparations together with teats in sterile wraps were made available for the general public. Because of cost it is not likely that these preparations will displace the powder formulations, but they will have an important role to play in providing night feeds, while travelling or in other circumstances when facilities for preparation of the normal formula feeds may not be available.

Over the last 10 years methods of preparing long-life products have been developed whereby highly perishable liquids, such as soups, milk and coffee whiteners, are preserved as aseptic 'long-life' liquids. The processes involve sterilization for a short time at a very high temperature followed by aseptic transfer to a sterile container under the protection of a blanket of sterile, often hot, inert gas, frequently with some further protection by an agent such as hydrogen peroxide. Vast numbers of these packs are now used every day, and range from 10 ml foil-capped plastic containers (for milk and coffee whiteners) to Tetrapaks and Combiblocs fabricated from metal–plastic–paper laminates up to 1 litre or even larger sizes. The success of these products in the retail market has encouraged the marketing in 1990 of RTF infant formulas in a laminated (paper–metal foil–plastic) heat-sealed pack similar to the smaller retail packs of fruit juices and milk now so common on the retail shelves.

Weaning foods

The young infant is immature in many ways: the gut, although adapted to a liquid diet, lacks the neuromuscular, digestive, absorptive and immunological characteristics needed for the use of adult diets (Milla, 1986). Weaning is the process during which the infant food is changed from a liquid regimen (breast or bottle) by incorporating increasing proportions of other items, notably solids. This process is usually initiated as the mother's supply of breast milk fails to keep pace with the growing infant's needs and ends as the child's developing physiology and teeth permit use of the family foods. Another important factor in many human groups may be the loss, after infancy, of the ability to digest lactose and hence the possibility of lactose intolerance.

The start of weaning, whether from breast or bottle, depends on a variety of circumstances. In Victorian times numerous cereal preparations were used for infant feeding either to make an infant food by adding cows' milk, or to be given during weaning as thicker gruels and porridges together with finely divided or sieved foods such as egg, meat, fish, vegetables or other cooked items. Barley water (made from pearl barley) was especially popular, as were gruels made from wheat and barley flours or from rolled oats. Such gruels normally contained less than 5% total solids, mainly carbohydrates, and were of only modest nutritional value (Dingwall-Fordyce, 1908). Other mixtures were used, e.g. proprietary farinaceous foods, pure starch (e.g. arrowroot and cornflour) as well as bread jelly (made by straining a preparation of toasted bread boiled in water). Some of these products, especially barley water and some herbal teas, were offered as drinks for thirsty infants. Mothers, then as now, seldom offered plain water. When water quality was questionable, dilute gruels and herb teas provided pathogen-free drinks in that they could only be made with hot water. Today herb-flavoured dry dextrose mixtures are sold for the preparation of 'soothing' drinks for infants by addition of water. These are presumably intended to replace, in convenient form, the 'soothing' and 'calming' herb teas of Victorian times.

In the 1890s and in the first decades of the present century, the usual advice was that weaning foods – sieved vegetables, meat and fish purées, fruit, puddings, cereals and semolina, for instance – should be introduced from the seventh to the eighth month, depending on circumstances (especially tooth eruption and bodily development). Introduction of these foods should be slow but progressive, with complete weaning from breast to bottle by the end of the first 12 months. Hard rusks and biscuits were often used to assist teething. Milk should still comprise a major proportion of the diet (Cautley, 1896, 1903; Cheadle, 1889, 1902; Hutchison, 1900–1906, Dingwall-Fordyce, 1908). Some proprietary manufactured cereal weaning foods were available in the late 19th and early 20th centuries, e.g. Allenburys malted food, Allenburys Rusks (Anon. 1898, 1911) and Farleys Rusks (Farley Health Foods), but these were expensive and limited in variety. For this reason, almost all weaning foods were made at home in the kitchen, from foods to be found in the larder!

From the 1890s to the 1920s the advice on weaning remained substantially unchanged. In 1921 a popular baby book advised initiation of weaning at 9 months and its completion at 12 months (Anon. 1921). This publication also emphasized the importance of milk even after weaning, and presented a series of recipes for the preparation, in the home, of numerous food items suitable for infants of varying ages (Anon. 1921). From about this time weaning practices began to change. Whitehead and Paul (1987) noted how, over the next few decades, the recommended weaning age and the age at which weaning was actually practised were both greatly reduced. One can only speculate as to why this trend may have occurred. It is possible that rising standards of living and improved kitchen facilities may have permitted the easier preparation of suitable foods in the home, while at the same time there was during this period emphasis on the benefits, especially for children, of a varied diet in overcoming the risk of nutritional, especially vitamin, deficiencies.

In the 1930s novel manufactured weaning foods became available to meet changing understanding of infant nutrition. These rapidly became popular because of their ease of preparation in the home and the then current belief that, being made under factory supervision, they would all in their different ways be of high hygienic and nutritional quality. This trend followed the publication by Tisdall *et al.* (1930) of laboratory and clinical trials to show the benefits to be attained by appropriate fortification of a cereal food with protein, vitamins and iron. These findings were applied in the UK to manufacture a precooked infant cereal food, which was not only very simple to prepare but which could also claim nutritional advantages over previous manufactured and home-made products (Anon. 1932).

In the 1930s a range of puréed foods in small cans and jars were made available for use as infant weaning foods. After the Second World War this range was considerably extended and their use greatly increased because of the convenience and reliability of these homogenized preparations of – among others – meats, fruits, cereals and made-up dishes (Anon. 1990).

After the Second World War the importance of a varied diet, especially for children, came to be generally appreciated. This may have encouraged variety, and hence additions to the diets of infants as well as children. Whatever the cause, recommendations were made in the 1950s to introduce cereals at $3\frac{1}{2}$ months and vegetable purées at 4 months (Anon. 1957). This tendency to wean early continued to develop during the 1960s, so that by 1967–1973 many infants were given cereals during the first month of life and 80–100% were given them by 3–4 months (DHSS, 1974). Indeed by 1973 one baby book, which had been approved by clinical consultants, specifically stated: 'When your baby is a few weeks old, or even a few days, if your doctor or clinic advises it, he may be introduced to foods besides milk . . .' (Anon. 1973). At that time it was said that 'the mothers often leave the clinics with a baby under one arm and a packet of Farex under the other'.

The belief in the 1960s that protein deficiency was a major cause of ill health (FAO/WHO, 1968) led to the marketing of protein-rich foods. Amongst these Farlene (Farley Health Products), marketed in 1962, was most successful in meeting the commonly accepted desirable features of a food, i.e. a variety of components and the presence of a high proportion of protein of good biological value.

The finding that infants were frequently subjected to needlessly high renal osmolar loads by excessive intakes of high-electrolyte milk formulas and weaning foods prompted action by the DHSS to advise changes in infant feeding practice in the UK. This was done by encouraging breast feeding, discouraging traditional high-electrolyte infant formulas and deprecating the early administration of weaning foods (DHSS, 1974). Later surveys (DHSS, 1988) show that this policy was successful in that the number of mothers breast feeding approximately doubled, from about 15% in 1980 to about 35% in 1985, while the infant milk formulas available after 1976 were all of the low-electrolyte type (Mettler, 1976, 1980a). However, the advice to delay the introduction of weaning foods does not appear to have been heeded as well as had been hoped, although the advice provided on manufactured weaning food preparations suggests weaning should begin at some time between the ages of 3 and 4 months. The DHSS (1988) also notes that cows' milk should continue to provide many of the nutrients needed by the young, weaned child, but that supplies of vitamin D and iron, in which cows' milk is deficient, should be assured from other sources. Alternatively a follow-up milk (as is frequently used in other countries) fortified with iron and vitamin D should be used in place of unmodified cows' milk.

REFERENCES

Anon. (1893) *New and Recent Remedies*, February, pp. 33–34. London: Allen & Hanbury.

Anon. (1898) *The Allenbury Foods for Infants* (Price list, section III), 14 October, pp. 87–89. London: Allen & Hanbury.

Anon. (1906) Allenburys on the Lee. *Chemist and Druggist*, 28 July, 134–137.

Anon. (1908) *The Glaxo Baby Book*. London: Joseph Nathan.

Anon. (1911) *General List of Drugs, Pharmaceuticals and the Allenburys Specialities* (section III), February, pp. 214, 216. London: Allen & Hanbury.

Anon. (1920) *Glaxo Service Bulletin*. 1 October (wrapper).

Anon. (1921) *The Glaxo Baby Book*. London: Joseph Nathan.

Anon. (1925) New style tin for Allenburys No. 1 and 2 Foods and Diet. *The Plough*, October, pp. 11–12. London: Allen & Hanbury.

Anon. (1932) Farex and cereal foods. *Nutrition*, 2(2), 25, 29–31.

Anon. (1953) Trade Notes. *Chemist and Druggist*, 27 June, 684.

Anon. (1957) *The Glaxo Handbook of Infant Nutrition*. Greenford: Glaxo.

Anon. (1973) *The Glaxo Mother and Baby Book*. Greenford: Glaxo.

Barber, H.J. and Page, J.E. (1982) T.S. Grimwade and the desiccated milk company. *Chemistry and Industry*, 352–353.

Barlow, T. (1894) Infantile scurvy and its relation to rickets. *Lancet*, ii, 1075–1080.

Barltrop, D. and Oppe, T.E. (1970) Dietary factors in neonatal calcium homeostasis. *Lancet*, ii, 1333–1335.

Barr, R.I. and Mettler, A.E. (1983) The artificial feeding of young infants in Britain. *Journal of the Royal Society of Health*, 4, 131–134.

Cautley, E. (1896) *The Natural and Artificial Methods of Feeding Infants and Young Children*. London: Churchill.

Cautley, E. (1903) *The Natural and Artificial Methods of Feeding Infants and Young Children*, 2nd edn. London: Churchill.

Central Statistical Office (1990) *Annual Abstract of Statistics, 1990* (edition no. 126). London: HMSO.

Cheadle, W.B. (1889) *Artificial Feeding of Infants, the Properties of Artificial Foods and the Diseases Arising from Faults of Diet in Early Life*. London: Smith Elder.

Cheadle, W.B. (1902) *Artificial Feeding of Infants, the Properties of Artificial Foods and the Diseases Arising from Faults of Diet in Early Life*, 5th edn. London: Smith Elder.

Codex Alimentarius Commission (1976) *Recommended International Standards for Foods for Infants and Children.* Rome: WHO/FAO.

Coutts, F.J.H. and Baker, J.L. (1914) *Reports to the Local Government Board on Public Health and Related Subjects.* New Series no. 80, Food Reports no. 20. London: HMSO.

Coward, E. (1985) *Gold on the Green.* Greenford: Glaxo.

Cuthbertson, W.F.J. (1963) Vitamin D activity of plasma in ideopathic hypercalcaemia. *Proceedings of the Nutrition Society*, 22, 146–153.

Cuthbertson, W.F.J. (1974) Infant food formulations. In *Milk Products of the Future*, pp. 51–59 (ed. J. Rothwell). Wembley: Society of Dairy Technology.

Cuthbertson, W.F.J. (1978) Nutritional aspects of milk products used for infant feeding. *Journal of the Society of Dairy Technology*, 31, 182–190.

Cuthbertson, W.F.J. (1982) Some applications of chemistry which improved the quality and availability of food over the last century. In *The Chemical Industry*, pp. 497–527 (eds D. Sharp and T.F. West). London: Society of Chemical Industry.

DHSS (UK) (1974) *Present Day Practice in Infant Feeding.* Reports on Health and Social Subjects no. 9. London: HMSO.

DHSS (UK) (1977) *The Composition of Mature Human Milk.* Reports on Health and Social Subjects no. 12. London: HMSO.

DHSS (UK) (1980a) *Artificial Feeds for the Young Infant.* Reports on Health and Social Subjects no. 18. London: HMSO.

DHSS (UK) (1980b) *Present Day Practice in Infant Feeding.* Reports on Health and Social Subjects no. 20. London: HMSO.

DHSS (UK) (1981) *The Collection and Storage of Human Milk.* Reports on Health and Social Subjects no. 22. London: HMSO.

DHSS (UK) (1988) *Present Day Practice in Infant Feeding, Third Report.* Reports on Health and Social Subjects no. 32. London: HMSO.

Dingwall-Fordyce, A. (1908) *Diet in Infancy.* London: William Green.

Dodd, W.R. (1892) British Patent no. 21 632. 13 February.

Drummond, J.C. and Wilbraham, A. (1939) *The Englishman's Food.* London: Jonathan Cape.

ESPGAN Committee on Nutrition (1977) *Acta Paediatrica Scandinavica* (Suppl. 262), 1–20.

FAO/WHO (1968) *International Action to Avert the Impending Protein Crisis.* Rome: WHO/FAO.

Farquharson, J., Cockburn, F., Patrick, W.A. *et al.* (1992) Infant cerebral cortex phospholipid fatty acid composition and diet. *Lancet*, 340, 810–813.

Fildes, V.A. (1986) *Breasts, Bottles and Babies.* London: Universal Press.

Fomon, S.J. (1967) *Infant Nutrition.* Philadelphia, PA: Saunders.

Hansen, A.E., Haggard, M.E., Boelsche, A.N. *et al.* (1958) *Journal of Nutrition*, 66, 565–576.

Hansen, A.E., Stewart, R.A., Highes, G. and Soderhjelm, L. (1962) The relation of linoleic acid to infant feeding. *Acta Paediatrica Scandinavica* (Suppl. 137), 1–41.

Hanson, L.A., Carlsson, B., Fallstrom, S.P. *et al.* (1982) Food and immunological development. *Acta Paediatrica Scandinavica* (Suppl. 299), 38–42.

Holman, R.T. (1972) Biological activities and requirements for polyunsaturated fatty acids. In *Progress in the Chemistry of Fats and Other Lipids*, vol. 10 (ed. R.T. Holman). Oxford: Pergamon Press.

Howarth, W.J. (1905) The influence of feeding on the mortality of infants. *Lancet*, ii, 210–213.

Hutchison, R. (1900–1956) *Food and Principles of Dietetics*, (1900, 1st edn; 1905, 2nd edn; 1906, 3rd edn; 1936, 8th edn; 1940, 9th edn; 1948, 10th edn; 1956, 11th edn). London: Edward Arnold.

IFA (USA) (1980) *Infant Formula Act*. Public law 96-359, 26 September.

Jephcott, H. (1969) *The First Fifty Years*. Greenford: Glaxo.

Jephcott, H. and Bacharach, A.L. (1921) The antiscorbutic value of dried milk. *Biochemical Journal*, 15, 129–139.

Jephcott, H. and Bacharach, A.L. (1926) A-rapid and reliable test for vitamin D. *Biochemical Journal*, 20, 1351–1355.

Jephcott, H. and Bacharach, A.L. (1928) The quantitative estimation of vitamin D. *Biochemical Journal*, 22, 60–62.

Kenny, J.E., Boesman, M.I. and Michaels, J.G. (1967) Bacterial and viral coprantibodies in breastfed infants. *Paediatrics*, 39, 202–213.

Kon, S.K. and Mawson, E.H. (1950) *Human Milk*. Special report to the Medical Research Council no. 269. London: HMSO.

Lightwood, R. and Stapleton, T. (1953) Idiopathic hypercalcaemia. *Lancet*, ii, 255–256.

Lovell, H.R. (1980) Fundamentals of spray drying. In *Milk and Whey Powders*, pp. 18–32 (ed. J. Rothwell). Wembley: Society of Dairy Technology.

Lucas, A., Morley, R., Cole, T.J. *et al.* (1992) Breast milk and subsequent intelligence quotient in children born preterm. *Lancet*, 339, 261–264.

McClelland, D.B.L., McGrath, J. and Samson, R.R. (1978) Antimicrobial factors in human milk. *Acta Paediatrica Scandinavica* (Suppl.), 271, 1–20.

MacKay, H.M. and Goodfellow, R. (1931) Medical Research Council Special Report Series no. 157. London: HMSO.

Macy, I.G., Kelly, H.J. and Sloan, R.E. (1953) *The Composition of Milks*. National Research Council Publication no. 254. Washington, DC: National Academy of Sciences.

Mettler, A.E. (1976) Infant milk powders compared on a common basis. *Postgraduate Medical Journal* (Suppl.), 8, 3–20.

Mettler, A.E. (1979) The application of whey products in the baby food industry. *Proceedings of the Institute of Food Science and Technology*, 12, 203–214.

Mettler, A.E. (1980a) Utilisation of whey products for infant feeding. *Journal of the Society of Dairy Technology*, 33, 67–72.

Mettler, A.E. (1980b) Chemical and physical aspects of whey quality. In *Milk and Whey Powders*, pp. 92–116 (ed. J. Rothwell). Wembley: Society of Dairy Technology.

Mettler, A.E. (1982) Infant formula. *Acta Paediatrica Scandinavica* (Suppl.) 299, 58–76.

Milla, P.J. (1986) The weanling gut. *Acta Paediatrica Scandinavica* (Suppl.), 323, 5–13.

Naish, A.E. (1908) The Sheffield Corporation scheme for reducing infant mortality. *The Medical Officer*, 5 September, 33–35.

Ogra, S.S., Weintraub, D. and Ogra, P.L. (1977) Immunological aspects of human colostrum and milk. III. Fate and absorption of cellular and soluble components in the gastrointestinal tract. *Journal of Immunology*, 119, 245–248.

Oppe, T.E. and Redstone, D. (1968) Calcium and phosphorus levels in healthy newborn infants given various types of milk. *Lancet*, i, 1045–1048.

Registrar General (1908) *Births, Marriages and Deaths for England and Wales for 1906*. Sixty-ninth Report of the Registrar General. London: HMSO.

Registrar General (1911) *Births, Marriages and Deaths for England and Wales for 1909*. Seventy-second Report of the Registrar General. London: HMSO.

Shaw, J.C.L., Jones, A. and Gunther, M. (1973) Mineral contents of brands of milk for infant feeding. *British Medical Journal*, **2**, 12–15.

Sheill, S. (1912) Epidemic gastro-enteritis. *The Practitioner*, **88**, 651–674.

Taitz, L.S. and Byers, H.D. (1972) High calorie osmolar feeding and hypertonic dehydration. *Archives of the Diseases of Children*, **47**, 257–260.

Tibbles, W. (1907) *Food and Hygiene* London: Rebman.

Tibbles, W. (1914) *Dietetics*. London: Ballière, Tyndall & Cox.

Tisdall, F.F., Drake, T.G.H. and Brown, A. (1930) A new cereal mixture containing vitamin and mineral elements. *American Journal of the Diseases of Children*, **40**, 791–799.

Warren, R.J. (1980) Packing and marketing of milk and whey powders. In *Milk and Whey Powders*, pp. 117–124 (ed. J. Rothwell). Wembley: Society of Dairy Technology.

Whitehead, R. and Paul, A. (1987) Changes in infant feeding practice in Britain during the last century. In *Infant Nutrition and Cardiovascular Disease*, pp. 1–10. Medical Research Council Environmental Epidemiology Unit Scientific Report no. 8.

Widdowson, E.M. and Spray, C.M. (1951) Chemical development in utero. *Archives of the Diseases of Children*, **26**, 205–214.

Widdowson, E.M., Chan, H., Harrison, G.E. and Milner, R.D.G. (1972) Accumulation of copper, zinc, manganese, chromium and cobalt in the human liver before birth. *Biology of the Neonate*, **20**, 360–367.

Willoughby, E.F. (1903) *Milk, its Production and Uses*. London: Griffin.

Wilson, G.S. (1942) *The Pasteurisation of Milk*. London: Edward Arnold.

Wilson, J.F. and Lahey, M.E. (1960) Failure to induce copper deficiency in premature infants. *Pediatrics*, **25**, 40–49.

Wulff, J. (1980) Instantizing milk and whey powders. In *Milk and Whey Powders*, pp. 33–48 (ed. J. Rothwell). Wembley: Society of Dairy Technology.

2
Nutrition during pregnancy: effects on the newborn

Jane B. Morgan
University of Surrey, Guildford, UK

INTRODUCTION

Pregnancy is a time of physiological stress to the mother primarily because of the increase in metabolism associated with the production of new tissue in the fetal membranes, fetus, placenta and mammary gland. A woman's diet prior to conception – indeed from her own conception – is now recognized as having an important impact on her ability to reproduce successfully. The theory that the intrauterine environment can have an important effect on the development of diet-related diseases in adult life has recently gained momentum. This has important implications for good nutrition and health of a girl throughout her life and the prevention of disease in the next generation.

This chapter will examine our knowledge concerning nutrition before and during pregnancy; special reference will be made to the effect of specific disorders (extremes of body weight, alcoholism, excessive caffeine consumption, atopic disease) and to less advantaged women (teenagers, situations of acute and chronic undernutrition). Beneficial effects to the newborn infant of supplementation in the maternal diet will also be chronicled. Finally the evidence for the influence of intrauterine nutrition and disease programming in future generations will be examined.

Infant Nutrition. Edited by A.F. Walker and B.A. Rolls.
Published in 1994 by Chapman & Hall, London.
ISBN 0 412 59140 5.

NUTRITION BEFORE CONCEPTION AND THE OUTCOME OF PREGNANCY

Chronically malnourished women living in marginal economic conditions have a high rate of miscarriage, yet this group may have a high rate of reproduction. Therefore to establish a relationship between maternal nutrition and the outcome of pregnancy is difficult and confounded by a number of variables. These may include food supply, access to medical care, level of education, cultural identity, previous experience with child rearing and earlier pregnancy experience. Both short-term and long-term maternal nutritional status are independently related to infant morbidity and mortality (Worthington-Roberts *et al.* 1985).

Nutrition can affect the duration of the reproductive life span. In the West the age of menarche is around 13 years (Johnston, 1974) whereas in developing countries there is a wider variation, but the age is generally later, e.g. 15 years in South African Bantu (Burrel and Tanner, 1961). Dreizen *et al.* (1967) in a study from the USA reported a 2-year delay in the onset of menarche in a group of poorly nourished girls compared with a group of well nourished girls. In Western society, marriage (and associated reproduction) generally occurs a number of years after the onset of menarche. However, in developing countries the two (menarche and marriage) can be closely linked, and in such societies an improvement in nutritional status (which would cause the age of menarche to fall) would have only a small impact on fertility.

The influence of nutrition on the menopause and thus reproductive outcome is less clear-cut. An undernourished woman may have an earlier menopause compared with her well nourished counterpart. However, the effect of malnutrition would only be important if it affected the timing of the last child born. This does not seem to be the case. Frish (1978) reports 40.9 and 41.7 years as the age of the mother giving birth to her last child in well nourished and undernourished women respectively.

The spacing of births has been considered in relation to the successful outcome of pregnancy. Close birth spacing increases the risk of miscarriage, congenital malformation and perinatal death because the mother does not have 'time to recover from nutritional depletion caused by the first pregnancy or time to recover a normal hormonal profile before the beginning of the next pregnancy' (Wynn, 1987). There is an optimum interval of 2–4 years between births. This interval may include the extension of amenorrhoea achieved by lactation. The onset of ovulation and menstruation in the lactating mother is delayed for at least 10 weeks (and usually much longer) provided breast feeding is complete, successful and unrestricted. Lactational amenorrhoea, however, is not a reliable contraceptive on an individual basis.

A study by Merchant *et al.* (1990) examined the consequences for maternal nutrition of reproductive stress across consecutive pregnancies in a large (over 1500 births) group of Guatemalan women. Data were analysed from records kept from 1971 to 1979. The Guatemalan data provided a rare opportunity to examine data on three consecutive pregnancies for each woman. Stress was assessed by examining responses in maternal supplement intake, maternal fat stores and birth weight. The supplement was liquid, contained (per 180 ml) 11 g protein and 682 kJ (163 kcal) and was offered to the women twice daily. The authors reported that overlap (lactation overlapping with pregnancy) and short recuperative intervals were related to increased supplement intake and reduced fat stores (i.e. stress). Birth weight of infants who were born at term was not affected, indicating that, at least in this group of women studied, fetal growth was being protected at the cost of maternal nutritional status. Such reports of nutrition and reproductive stress lead onto the question, how serious does nutritional deprivation have to be before the outcome of pregnancy is compromised?

The extreme hardship of the Second World War provided an opportunity to study the effects of severe (or chronic) dietary restriction before conception and during pregnancy on the fetus under conditions unlikely to be duplicated. The Dutch famine lasted for approximately 6 months during the winter of 1944. The daily dietary intakes of the women were reported to be about 4.18 MJ (1000 kcal) and 30–40 g protein. Because of the timing of the famine its effect could be compared on infants conceived before and during food shortage. Figure 2.1 illustrates the high incidence of still births after the famine was over among infants who had been conceived during the hungry winter. Congenital malformations were highest in infants conceived during the famine, and lowest in infants conceived before it. Those infants who were conceived and who survived the famine weighed on average 200 g less than infants conceived before the onset of famine. Birth weights were lowest in infants exposed to famine during the later stages of pregnancy. Those infants who were exposed to famine in the first and second trimester of pregnancy had higher birth weights than those exposed only during the last 3 weeks of gestation (Smith, 1947).

MATERNAL VITAMIN STATUS AND MALFORMATIONS OF THE NEURAL TUBE

Over the last 20 years evidence has been accumulating that there may be a nutritional component in the environmental contribution to defects of the neural tube, anencephalus and spina bifida. These malformations are amongst the commonest reported in the UK, affecting one to five per 1000 babies, and a substantial number of spontaneously aborted fetuses.

Still births per 1000 total births

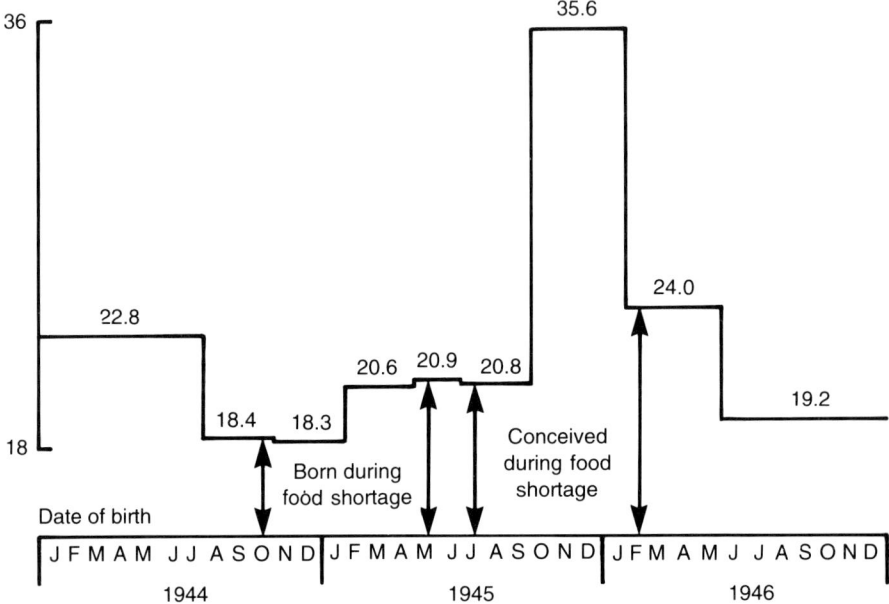

Figure 2.1 Food shortage and still birth, babies born or conceived through the 'Dutch Hunger Winter' 1944–1945 (154 365 births). (Reproduced with permission from Wynn, 1987.)

Although a small number of neural tube defects (NTD) have a purely genetic basis, the great majority result from an interaction between genetic and environmental factors. Rates are high in the Irish, low in those of Afro-Caribbean origin, high in Sikhs and low in other Indian ethnic groups. Many environmental factors have been considered, including infection, soft water, the consumption of blighted potatoes, and poor nutrition, specifically related to vitamin intake (particularly the B group). The association between poor nutritional status and NTD has recently been reviewed by Schorah and Smithells (1991). It is of interest that NTD incidence is relatively low in areas of endemic protein–energy malnutrition.

A role for certain micronutrients, vitamin A, zinc and folic acid, has been suggested in the causation of NTD in man. There have been reports of increased prevalence of NTD in women who have received gastric bypass surgery, and these women often have low serum B_{12} and folic acid concentrations.

NTD arises very early in fetal life (about the 4th week) and therefore nutritional status during this time (peri-conceptual nutrition) has evoked the greatest interest. A recent intervention trial (cited by Schorah and Smithells, 1991) was undertaken to evaluate whether multivitamin supplements would reduce the recurrence rate of NTD in women of high risk. These women have approximately 10-fold higher risk of recurrence of NTD than the general population.

Volunteers were asked to take the supplement for not less than 28 days before conception, and to continue into well after the time of the neural tube closure. The supplement provided most vitamins (including folic acid, but not vitamin B_{12}), iron and calcium (but not zinc). Table 2.1 indicates a clear reduction in the rate of NTD in those mothers who took the vitamin supplement. This study and others cited by Schorah and Smithells (1991) indicate a protective effect of folic acid in very early pregnancy. Schorah and Smithells (1991) speculate that diet would alter the supply of nutrients, and genetic factors alter the metabolism of nutrients, thus leading to reduced nutrient provision to the embryo, the two interacting to affect neural tube closure. Experimental evidence exists for such an interaction, particularly with regard to folic acid. There is also epidemological evidence. An increased frequency of NTD among women receiving vitamin supplements in areas with a low prevalence of NTD can be accounted for by the possibility that women responsive to vitamin supplements already have adequate nutrient intakes. Unresponsive women may have metabolic problems that are not responsive to supplementation, or require supraphysiological doses.

Ideally, supplements should be given from 28 days pre-conception. In future a screening test should be developed that would identify the metabolic lesion associated to NTD and prevent unnecessary supplementation of very large numbers of women.

Table 2.1 Results of intervention study investigating the effect of nutrient supplementation of women before and after conception on the incidence of neural tube defect (NTD) in their infants

		No. of NTD cases	
	Normal	*Found*	*Expected*[a]
Fully supplemented	426	3	20
Unsupplemented	486	24	24

From Schorah and Smithells (1991).
Number of NTD was significantly different with the supplemented compared with the unsupplemented group ($P < 0.01$, Fisher's exact test).
[a]Assumes 4% recurrence rate after one previous NTD, 10% after two NTD cases.

Thus a picture emerges that poor nutrition in the early months affects embryonic development and survival; in the later stages poor nutrition affects fetal growth.

DIETS IN PREGNANCY AND RECOMMENDATIONS OF NUTRIENT INTAKE

Over the last decade our understanding of what women actually eat in pregnancy and how this relates to requirements has made great progress. A five-country (Scotland, the Netherlands, the Gambia, Thailand and the Philippines) integrated study was undertaken to resolve the debate regarding the energy cost of pregnancy (Durnin, 1987). Results (Table 2.2) indicated that energy intakes did not remotely conform to the theoretical expected quantities of the energy cost of pregnancy (Table 2.3). These theoretical calculations of the energy cost over the course of pregnancy (355 MJ, 85 000 kcal; Hytten and Chamberlain, 1980) have been used as the basis for international recommendations (Table 2.3). Furthermore, the FAO/WHO/UNU (1985) report indicated that the extra daily energy cost (amounting to 1.2 MJ, 285 kcal) should be derived from increased food consumption. However, the results from the integrated study throw new light on the picture. In this study the energy cost of pregnancy was estimated to be about 250 MJ (60 000 kcal). However, this cost was not reflected in an extra 250 MJ being consumed in the diet throughout pregnancy (Durnin, 1987); the additional intake was reported to be no more than 118 MJ (28 000 kcal) or 420 kJ (100 kcal) daily. This

Table 2.2 Some characteristics of the mother and her infant from the integrated five-country study

	Scotland	The Netherlands	The Gambia	Thailand	The Philippines
No. of mothers	88	57	52	44	51
Age (years)	28	28	26	23	23
Weight (kg)	57	63	51	48	44
Height (m)	1.6	1.7	1.6	1.5	1.5
Daily energy intake[a]					
(MJ)	8.9	8.9	–	8.0	7.3
(kcal)	2130	2130	–	1915	1745
Birth weight (g)	3370	3458	2980	2980	2885

From Durnin (1987).
[a]Measurement at or near 10 weeks gestation.

Table 2.3 Recommended intakes of food energy and protein and nutrients relating to non-pregnant and pregnant women. Values per day unless otherwise stated

	FAO/WHO (1985)		NRC (USA) (1989)	
	Non-pregnant	*Pregnant*	*Non-pregnant*	*Pregnant*
Weight (kg)	55	67.5	58	70.5
Weight gain (kg)	–	12.5	–	12.5
Total energy				
(MJ)	8.8[a]	9.9	9.2	10.5[b]
(kcal)	2100	2385	2200	2500
Total cost of pregnancy				
(MJ)	–	335	–	210
(kcal)	–	80 000	–	50400
Protein (g)	41	47	46	60
Vitamin D (µg)	–	–	10	10
Folacin (mg)	–	–	180	400
Vitamin B_{12} (mg)	–	–	2.0	2.2
Calcium (mg)	–	–	1200	1200
Iron (mg)	–	–	15	30

[a] Basal metabolic rate × 1.6.
[b] Second and third trimesters only.

implies that there are mechanisms involving the conservation of energy, and that enhanced efficiency of energy metabolism is occurring together with subtle changes in activity levels (Fig. 2.2).

A Swedish study by Forsum *et al.* (1988) examined resting metabolic rate, body composition and energy requirement in 22 healthy pregnant women. Resting rate increased during pregnancy and was positively correlated to birth weight. Fat gain was 5.8 kg, 60% of which had already been gained by 16–18 weeks' gestation. However, gain was unrelated to birth weight. The authors speculate that a 'factor' associated with maternal lean body mass (and not fat) could be associated with the infant's birth weight. All variables in this study had wide standard deviations, and this fact together with an apparent lack of accord with similar studies on well nourished pregnant women indicate the difficulty in estimating energy requirements for a hypothetical pregnant woman. The practical consequence of this has been highlighted by Prentice *et al.* (1989), who demonstrated a very high degree of variation in the individual energy cost of pregnancy, with estimates ranging from −16 to 276 MJ (−3825–66 000 kcal; coefficient of variation 93%). This variation makes the task of recommending energy requirements for individual women

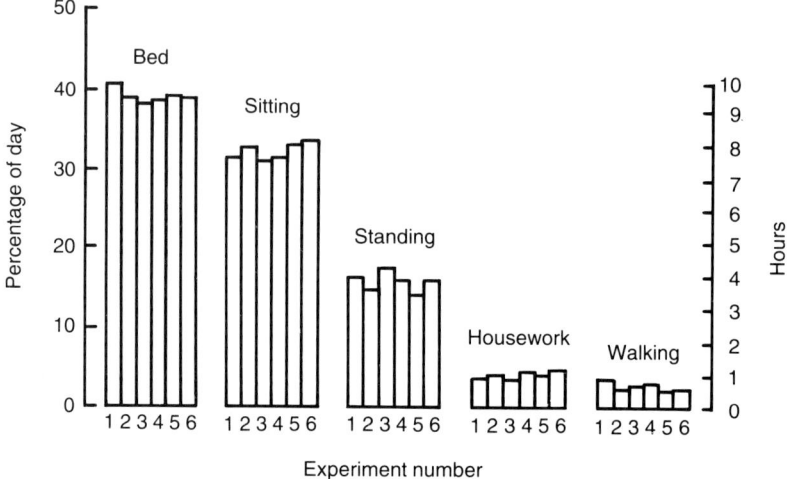

Figure 2.2 Duration of different activities at six periods throughout pregnancy. Period 1 at 8–12 weeks, other periods followed at 6-week intervals. (Reproduced with permission from Durnin *et al.*, 1987.)

extremely difficult. Moreover, the adaptive responses may represent a 'powerful selection trait, since neonatal mortality is clearly correlated to infant birth weight, and since the mother's ability to adopt energy-sparing mechanisms may help to prevent intrauterine growth retardation when dietary energy is scarce' (Prentice *et al.* 1989).

Comprehensive data on intakes of the proximate nutrients and vitamins and minerals in similar detail from different countries are lacking. However, there is information of between-region (UK) dietary intakes from 265 pregnant and non-pregnant women in different social groups living in London or Edinburgh with respect to calcium, iron, retinol, ascorbic acid and folic acid (Schofield *et al.* 1989). There were no consistent trends regarding the pattern of intakes of the micronutrients studied. Mean intakes of calcium and iron were reported to be below the then current UK recommended daily amount (RDA; DHSS, 1979), whereas overall intakes of retinol were above the RDA, and ascorbic acid intakes ranged above and below the RDA. Reported intakes of folic acid revealed that the London mean values were consistently higher than those in Edinburgh, and that intakes favoured social classes 1 and 2 (professional and managerial people). All mean intakes of folic acid were 50% below the US RDA. Folate supplements were commonly used (e.g. 82% of the London group), although supplement contribution was not included in the data analysis. All 265 mothers produced healthy babies, and none seemed to be clinically nutritionally deficient.

EXTREMES IN BODY WEIGHT IN THE MOTHER

Tall and heavy mothers have, on average, babies who weigh up to 500 g more at birth compared with babies of short and light mothers. This phenomenon is not influenced to any extent by the size of the father (Worthington-Roberts *et al.* 1985). However, excessive ranges in body weight (obesity or leanness) at the time of conception are both contra-indicated for the successful outcome of pregnancy in terms of the health of the mother and the effect on her baby. Table 2.4 provides information of the incidence of low birth weight infants derived from a study under-taken in the USA on just under 4000 women divided into three weight classes. These data may mask the risks associated with excessive obesity in the mother at the onset of pregnancy to both herself and the infant. Using the index of low birth weight incidence together with other indicators, further evidence of the disadvantage of low pre-pregnancy weight can be seen in Table 2.5. Weight gain during pregnancy has a profound influence on infant birth weight and is the most important correlate of all variables. A study on 10 000 births revealed that women who gained less than 6.8 kg had more low birth weight infants than women who gained more than 16 kg (Table 2.6).

The evidence would indicate therefore that maternal underweight and poor weight gain during pregnancy have a profound impact on infant morbidity. Certainly dietary restriction is not advisable. Indeed those women who deliberately restrict their dietary intake during pregnancy to guarantee a quick return to their pre-pregnancy figure should be actively discouraged from doing so.

Many obstetricians today, especially in the USA, still advocate that pregnant women should eat less and therefore gain less weight, thereby reducing the risk of pregnancy toxaemia. There is obviously no such

Table 2.4 Incidence of low birth weight infants of women of different weights at pregnancy onset in the USA (3939 white mothers)

Weight at pregnancy onset (height adjusted)	Percentage of infants with birth weight under 2500 g
Heaviest 10%	2.3
Middle 10%	4.2
Lightest 10%	7.8

Cited from Morgan (1988).

Table 2.5 Infant morbidity in underweight and normal weight women, expressed as percentage of total births

Infant morbidity	Low pre-pregnancy weight	Normal weight controls
Low birth weight	15.3	7.6
Prematurity	23.0	14.0
Low Apgar score[a]	19.0	12.0

From Worthington-Roberts *et al.* (1985).
[a]Apgar: see Whitelaw (1991). This score is used as a developmental check and is, for example, the most common method of recording the degree of hypoxia at birth.

Table 2.6 Mothers' weight gain in pregnancy and the percentage of infants with low birth weight

Pregnancy weight gain of mother (kg)	Percentage of infants born under 2500 g
16.4+	3.0
11.8–16.4	4.3
7.3–11.7	8.2
0–6.8	15.2

Cited from Morgan (1988).

justification for such restrictions in the present day's climate of technical expertise in the labour unit.

MATERNAL ATOPIC DISEASE AND EFFECTS ON THE NEWBORN

Immunological development occurs early in intrauterine life and at birth an infant has an immune system similar to that of adults, although it has not developed in response to specific antigens. In the normal course of events tolerance develops, and the capacity of an individual to react to a normally effective antigenic stimulus (e.g. food protein) is established. Development of oral tolerance is associated with specific T-cells and affected by specifically activated T-suppressor cells (Bruce and Ferguson, 1986).

Hypersensitivity occurs when the secondary boosting of the immune response to an antigen is excessive and leads to gross tissue damage manifested as asthma, oedema and urticaria. In normal circumstances T-cells are able to evaluate the threat posed by an antigen and can distinguish between harmless and harmful antigens. When the system breaks down harmless substances are thought to be harmful, thereby provoking an immune response. Food hypersensitivity reactions are generally type I, anaphylactic, or type III, complex-mediated reactions (Brostoff, 1987). An example of type I hypersensitivity is atopic disease, classically characterized by familial predisposition.

Atopic disease is related to a number of risk factors, including race, gender, maternal age, family structure, lifestyle and environmental factors, in particular early feeding history. The strongest predisposing factor to the development of atopic disease is, however, family history, with the risk of developing allergy 10% if neither parent is atopic, 50% if one parent is atopic, and 66% if both parents are atopic (Bleumink, 1983).

Little is known regarding the complexity of the immunological response to the first eaten antigens in the vulnerable, relatively immune-deficient infant. However, the search to find a means of delaying, controlling or preventing infantile atopic disease has recently centred on diet. The concept that manipulation of maternal dietary intake during pregnancy and lactation to exclude allergenic food proteins may influence the progression of atopic disease in the infant was put forward by Cant *et al.* (1986) and Lovegrove *et al.* (1990). Because it has been known for some time that certain food proteins (egg, cows' milk) are detectable in breast milk, the exclusion of these proteins from the mother's diet might protect infants with a family history of atopic disease from developing eczema (Cant *et al.* 1986). Results from two controlled studies on 37 breast-fed infants with eczema indicated that there was benefit to some breast-fed infants with eczema.

The possibility that maternal dietary exclusion during pregnancy may evoke similar benefits to the potentially vulnerable fetus has recently been investigated (Lovegrove *et al.* 1990). In her study three groups of women were recruited: a control (non-atopic) group, an atopic group and a group of women who followed a milk-free diet in the last 6 weeks of pregnancy. Subjects on the exclusion diet were provided with a hypoallergic formula (Pepti-Junior, Cow & Gate, Trowbridge) to consume in the place of milk and milk products. Table 2.7 illustrates the biochemical results relating to two antibodies, to β-lactoglobulin and α-casein, in the maternal serum and fetal cord blood. The authors reported a strong positive relationship between maternal serum levels of β-lactoglobulin IgG and cord blood levels of the same antibody. Levels of β-lactoglobulin IgG were significantly higher in fetal cord blood compared with levels in maternal blood for the atopic and control groups, which implies the presence of a positive transport system for IgG antibodies. Both dietary restriction and the presence of atopic disease had an effect on IgG antibody levels. Mothers who followed the milk-free diet had significantly lower levels of β-lactoglobulin IgG than when they were not following the diet. The levels of both α-casein IgG and β-lactoglobulin IgG in atopic mothers were higher

Table 2.7 Effect of milk-free diet on mean maternal and fetal cord blood milk antibody levels (μg/ml) in control (non-atopic) and atopic pregnant women, and in women following a milk-free diet in late pregnancy

Group: No. in group:	Control 10	Atopic 10	Milk-free diet 9[a]
β-Lactoglobulin IgG			
Predelivery serum	30.2	50.8	88.7
Cord serum	36.8[c]	62.2[c]	88.9
Diet serum[b]	–	–	74.0[d]
α-Casein IgG			
Predelivery serum	12.6	30.4	64.6
Cord serum	14.3	25.5	46.0
Diet serum[b]	–	–	63.2

From Lovegrove *et al.* (1990).
[a]Seven atopic, two non-atopic women.
[b]Serum obtained from mothers when following the milk-free diet.
[c]Significantly higher ($P < 0.01$) than in maternal blood.
[d]Significantly lower ($P < 0.05$) than when these women were not following the diet.

(35%) than levels in non-atopic control subjects. The authors concluded that milk IgG antibodies in fetal cord blood were dependent on maternal levels, and that a milk-free diet in pregnancy can reduce both maternal and fetal levels of IgG. The results of this study suggest that pregnant women who have a family history of atopic disease should consider dietary restriction of selected food proteins. This course of action may minimize the effect of potential high levels of exposure of IgG antibodies to the fetus who has a compromised immune system, and thus delay the possibility of sensitization to food proteins in infancy.

MATERNAL ALCOHOL CONSUMPTION AND EFFECTS ON THE NEWBORN

There is no doubt that pregnancy and alcohol do not mix. Historical evidence has indicated that alcoholic mothers often give birth to infants with malformations. At this extreme end of alcohol abuse where a woman may be consuming more than 2 g of alcohol per kilogram body weight per day during gestation (particularly in the early stages of pregnancy) her offspring will develop what has now become known as the 'fetal alcohol syndrome' (FAS). This is characterized by a pattern of abnormalities which includes prenatal and postnatal growth deficiency, developmental delay, microcephaly, short palpebral fissures, maxillary hypoplasia and joint anomalies (Wright, 1988). The incidence of FAS can range from one in 300 live births to one in 2000 live births depending on the population studied. Poor nutrition and the use of drugs are often associated with alcoholism. Nutritional deficiencies are associated with poor fetal growth: there are reports of low zinc status, which may complicate the effects of alcoholism, causing congenital defects.

There are contraindications for the consumption of alcohol in women of childbearing age who may be considered as social drinkers or moderate consumers of alcohol (less than 1 g ethanol per kilogram body weight per day). This practice, particularly if reported around the time of conception or in the very early stages of pregnancy, may adversely affect intrauterine growth. Data from various sources have indicated that birth weight can be reduced by 3 g for every 1 g pure ethanol consumed in early pregnancy (Little, 1977) or could be so serious as to retard intrauterine growth by 1% for every 10 g alcohol consumed per day during pregnancy.

The first question is therefore whether there is a 'safe limit' of alcohol consumption at conception and during pregnancy. Second, there is a question regarding infrequent binge drinking, and whether this practice has the same adverse effects as consistent and habitual drinking. The effects of alcohol and smoking in pregnancy are synergic. Excessive maternal smoking accompanied by either heavy or moderate drinking has resulted in more pronounced deficits in fetal neurological development than heavy drinking alone. There is clear evidence therefore that women should be encouraged to attend pre-conceptional clinics where they should be advised to abstain from smoking and reduce their intake of alcohol to less than 100 g (10 drinks) per week. Total abstinence would be ideal. In the later stages of pregnancy detrimental effects on the fetus are less apparent, and in this case the mother should be advised accordingly.

The mode of action of the toxic effect of alcohol is not well understood. Alcohol passes freely across the placental barrier, and it is possible that ethanol exerts a direct teratogenic effect on the developing embryo in early pregnancy. Alternatively, acetaldehyde may constitute the primary toxin. There is also a possibility that alcohol-induced hypoglycaemia may cause central nervous system dysfunction to which the fetus is susceptible.

One objective for the future must be to establish a level of maternal alcohol consumption below which there would be no embryotoxic or teratogenic effects of alcohol or its derivatives. It may be that the recommended safe level would vary during the course of pregnancy, so that at conception and in the first trimester no alcohol should be consumed, in the second trimester 0.1 g/kg body weight per day would be the safe limit and in the third trimester 0.5 g/kg body weight daily would be considered to be a safe limit for consumption.

MATERNAL CAFFEINE CONSUMPTION AND EFFECTS ON THE NEWBORN

Caffeine is present in many drinks (coffee, tea, carbonated drinks) and in drugs used for allergies and colds. Graham (1978) has estimated that three-quarters of pregnant women in the USA consume caffeine, with a mean intake of two cups per day. Caffeine diffuses freely across the placental barrier, and concentrations are slightly lower in the embryonic tissue than those in maternal plasma (Driscoll *et al.* 1990).

Studies have shown that women who consume excessive amounts of coffee during pregnancy (more than five cups a day) are more likely to have premature labour, a small-for-gestational-age infant and a higher than average incidence of impending abortion (Furuhashi *et al.* 1985). In addition, there is evidence that excessive maternal caffeine consumption has a detrimental effect on fetal bone weight and calcium content. A recent study by Driscoll *et al.* (1990) examined the prenatal effects of maternal caffeine intake and high dietary protein on mandibular development in fetal rats. The caffeine supplement was equivalent to a daily intake of 10 cups of coffee in a 50 kg woman. Results from the study (Table 2.8) indicate that the effect of caffeine on the mandible in the rat fetus is altered by maternal dietary protein intake and that a high level of protein intake can 'buffer' the effect of caffeine. Thus an interaction between maternal caffeine intake and dietary protein levels during pregnancy may be important to bone development in fetal life, which implies that the effects of caffeine may be modified by different nutritional conditions.

Although caution must always be exercised in extrapolation from animal work to humans, pregnant women are nevertheless frequently exposed to caffeine, and the increased consumption of carbonated drinks

Table 2.8 Effects of caffeine supplementation and protein intake on characteristics in rats (mean values)

	Body weight (g)	Mandibular weight (mg)	Alkaline phosphatase activity (IU/mg protein)
200 g protein/kg diet			
No supplement	7.0	4.85	0.982
Caffeine supplement	6.4	4.13	0.582
400 g protein/kg diet			
No supplement	7.4	5.04	0.307
Caffeine supplement	6.8	4.96	0.872

From Driscoll *et al.* (1990).

containing caffeine indicates that caffeine consumption in pregnant women is increasing and may be a cause for concern.

HYPERTENSION AND PRE-ECLAMPSIA IN PREGNANCY

The diagnosis of mild pre-eclampsia in pregnancy is traditionally based on a blood pressure reading of (140/90 mmHg), proteinuria and oedema in the 20th week of gestation, or both. The incidence of pre-eclampsia reported from a survey conducted in Scotland was 24% and 10% in primigravidae and multigravidae respectively. Disorders relating to hypertension in pregnancy can be defined as follows (Gant and Worley, 1980).

A. Pregnancy-induced hypertension
   1. Pre-eclampsia
      (a) mild
      (b) severe
   2. Eclampsia
B. Chronic hypertension preceding pregnancy (any aetiology)
C. Chronic hypertension (any aetiology with superimposed pregnancy-induced hypertension)
D. Late or transient hypertension
   'Toxaemia' is no longer considered an appropriate term in this context; no toxin has ever been identified.

In the past, dietary management has involved a regimen restricted in protein to 45–60 g/day and restricted in sodium to 0.5 g/day, together with weight control.

The pathogenesis of pregnancy-induced hypertension has not been elucidated but is almost certainly multifactorial, with immunological, hormonal and nutritional influences. Until recently, the nutritional factors implicated from epidemiological, clinical and laboratory studies have included intakes of protein, salt and vitamin B_6.

More recently attention has focused on the role of essential fatty acids (Gant and Worley, 1980), in particular those in fish oils, in relation to early delivery and pre-eclampsia (Olsen and Secher, 1990). This latter study was based on a trial conducted more than 50 years ago by the People's League of Health, in which more than 5000 women were recruited to assess the effects of dietary supplement consisting of vitamins, minerals and halibut liver oil. The authors claim that the trial, conducted in London, is the only controlled trial in which fish oil has been given to pregnant women. (A control group received no supplement.) The supplement, provided from the 20th week of gestation, contained among other nutrients halibut liver oil, providing 5.6 mg retinol and 0.0225 mg cholecalciferol. The amount of eicosapentaenoic acid plus docosahexaenoic acid provided by the halibut liver oil was estimated to be about 0.1 g/day. The daily intake of *n*–3 fatty acids in pregnant women in London today is approximately 0.2 g. Re-evaluation of the data from this large trial revealed that in the supplemented group there was a reduction of 20.4% in the odds of delivering before 40 weeks gestational age and a reduction of 31.5% in the development of pre-eclampsia, compared with the control group. This impressive effect could not be explained by the vitamin or mineral supplement, as more recent trials had failed to show that they had any preventive effects on pre-eclampsia and early delivery. Why should marine fish oils have such an effect? One explanation may be that *n*–3 fatty acids down-regulate the arachidonic acid-derived prostaglandins that are mediators of labour. The preventive effect of *n*–3 fatty acids on pre-eclampsia is thought to be mediated in part via an inhibitor of the production of pro-platelet aggregatory and vasoconstrictory thromboxane A_2. The biochemical mechanisms involved need to be elucidated, and a controlled trial that assesses the isolated effects of fish oil is warranted.

PREGNANCY, NUTRITION AND THE ADOLESCENT

The pregnant adolescent can vary to a great extent in her physiological maturity and social circumstances; each individual represents a challenge. There is no doubt, however, that many young women who conceive during adolescence will have completed growing (approximately 4 years post menarche) and do not differ greatly in nutritional requirements from their adult counterparts. The group that is potentially the most vulnerable comprises those who become pregnant while still growing (2 years or less post menarche).

It has often been hypothesized that there is competition for nutrients between the still growing pregnant adolescent and her fetus (Naeye, 1981). Birth weight is, for obvious reasons, the most frequently used indicator of successful pregnancy outcome and reflects, if somewhat crudely, the nutritional status *in utero*. Much attention has been paid recently to maternal weight gain during pregnancy, birth weight and maternal growth (Stevens-Simon and McAnarney, 1988; Hediger *et al.* 1990; Scholl *et al.* 1990).

Maternal weight gain is one of the most important independent predictors of birth weight. In the USA in 1982 13.8% of infants born to women less than 15 years old weighed less than 2500 g compared with 5.8% of infants born to women 15–19 years old. As a result of this, some authorities have recommended that very young pregnant adolescents should gain much more weight during pregnancy than the 9–14 kg usually recommended (Hytten and Chamberlain, 1980). Caution was advised by Stevens-Simons and McAnarney (1988) 'because the mechanisms underlying the interaction between maternal age and weight gain are incompletely understood, and may include such diverse factors as incomplete maternal growth, reproductive immaturity, diminished maternal body size, nutritional deficiencies, socioeconomic and behavioural factors *and* maternal emotional stress'. A study by Hediger *et al.* (1990) provided some insight into the subject of optimum weight gain during adolescent pregnancy (subjects aged 15–18 years) and birth weight. They reported that the median weight gain at term (14.2–15.5 kg) was significantly greater than that reported for fully mature pregnant women, and that weight velocity was greater from the beginning of pregnancy in adolescent pregnancy compared with adult pregnancy. The authors speculated that these findings may be important in ensuring that the mother has sufficient reserves to support rapid fetal growth in the latter stages of pregnancy. Table 2.9 illustrates birth weight outcome by pre-pregnancy body mass index (BMI) and weight gain.

There is no doubt that continuing maternal growth is inexorably linked to the competition for nutrients between the mother and her fetus. Recently, in an elegant study by Scholl *et al.* (1990), an association was found between maternal growth (using the ingenious knee-height measuring device) and infant birth weight in multiparous adolescents (Fig. 2.3).

The knee-height measuring device was incorporated into the study as a means of assessing maternal growth as all gravidas shrink during the course of pregnancy (0.5 cm over 6 months). In those mothers (mean age

Table 2.9 Birth weight[a] (g) outcome by pre-pregnancy weight and weight gain

| Weight gain | Pre-pregnancy weight | | |
	Underweight	Normal weight	Overweight
<25th percentile			
Hispanics	3063 (59)[b]	3209 (47)	3330 (10)
Blacks	2938 (79)	3026 (77)	3173 (43)
Whites	3135 (57)	3306 (62)	3410 (17)
25–75th percentiles			
Hispanics	3226 (68)	3355 (56)	3043 (12)
Blacks	3263 (69)	3209 (119)	3347 (23)
Whites	3418 (120)	3353 (89)	3355 (18)
>75th percentile			
Hispanics	3211 (15)	3384 (20)	3349 (8)
Blacks	3187 (20)	3286 (31)	3207 (32)
Whites	3503 (54)	3505 (69)	3587 (21)

From Hediger *et al.* (1990).
[a]Least-square means of birth weight from a three-way analysis of covariance, blocking by ethnicity, pre-pregnancy weight, and weight gain and adjusting for length of gestation, maternal age, height, parity and smoking.
[b]Numbers of subjects in parentheses.

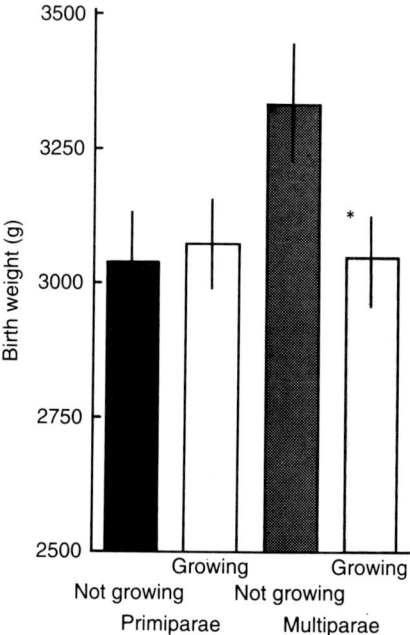

Figure 2.3 Effects of maternal growth in knee height on birth weight of infants. *Significant difference (*P* < 0.05) in birth weights (282 g) between infants of non-growing and growing multiparas after controlling for length of gestation, black ethnicity, age, maternal height, pre-pregnant body mass index and smoking. (Reproduced with permission from Scholl *et al.*, 1990.)

15.7 years) in whom knee-height growth was recorded during a subsequent adolescent pregnancy, there was a significant decrease (282 g) in birth weight as compared with infants whose mothers were not still growing. The fact that no such association was demonstrable in primiparas is of interest, and may be explained by the good nutritional status in this group. The authors speculated that competition for nutrients between the mother and her fetus in primigravidas may be more apparent in young mothers in less developed countries with all the biological and social problems associated with that lifestyle.

Two important questions remain unanswered. The optimal weight gain for pregnant adolescents is still being argued, and it is not known whether pregnancy at a low gynaecological age interferes with further maternal growth and development.

MATERNAL NUTRITIONAL STATUS AND FETAL GROWTH

Over the past 20 years there have been a number of intervention or supplementation trials that have reported on the effectiveness or otherwise of improved maternal nutrition on subsequent birth weight. The results of a number of these trials have been reviewed by Morgan (1988). It was apparent from these studies that a lack of energy rather than protein was the factor most likely to limit fetal growth. There is a threshold of daily maternal nutrient intake, around 7 MJ (1680 kcal), below which intervention would seem to benefit the outcome of pregnancy. A second factor that emerged from the earlier trials was that the effectiveness of supplementation on birth weight was disappointing, and it was noteworthy that marginally nourished mothers have infants whose birth weights persistently remain below those of infants born in Europe and the USA. Supplementation is nutritionally costly: an extra 42 MJ (10 000 kcal) consumed in pregnancy achieves increases in birth weight of only 25–84 g; thus it has become apparent that food supplementation should be targeted to those women most at risk. Unless a women is either on the edge of negative energy balance, or indeed in negative energy balance, supplementation may prove ineffectual.

As most of the early studies investigating undernourished women receiving dietary supplements have shown only minor positive effects on the outcome of pregnancy (usually defined as increase in birth weight), and many early trials had procedural flaws (Susser, 1981), recent studies have selected target groups more carefully. It is, however, established that underweight mothers who gain little weight during pregnancy are at great risk of producing an intrauterine growth-retarded infant, an effect that can be reversed if weight gain is improved. Two recent studies, one conducted in Chile (Mardones-Santander *et al.* 1988) and one in East Java (Kardjati *et al.* 1990), have thrown further light on the subject, by the target selection of a group of women likely to benefit from supplementation, by the use of appropriate supplements, and by monitoring the amount of supplement consumed and investigating variables previously not considered (e.g. pre-pregnancy weight). In the Chilean study, conducted from June 1983 to March 1984 in a low-income area in Santiago, a subject was selected only if she was found to be underweight and to meet the other enrolment criteria. Subjects were provided with one of two supplements, either a powdered milk (Purita®, PUR) or a powdered milk-based fortified product (Vita Nova Motherfood, VN).

Table 2.10 gives results of the outcome of the trial for those women who remained in the trial. This study was of particular interest as the non-compliers were identified and the outcome of their pregnancies described.

Table 2.10 Outcome of pregnancy in two groups of Chilean women given one of two dietary supplements (mean values)

| | Supplement given | |
	Milk power	Milk-based fortified product
No. of women in group	391	391
Gestational age at delivery (weeks)	39	39
Birth weight (g)	3105	3178*
Birth length (cm)	49	49
Head circumference (cm)	34	34
Intrauterine growth retardation (%)	43	32*
Birth weight < 2001 g (%)	9	6
Birth weight < 3001 g (%)	40	32*

From Mardones-Santander *et al.* (1988).
*Differences between the groups were statistically significant ($P < 0.05$).

The study lacked a randomly assigned unsupplemented group, which makes it difficult to draw any conclusions regarding absolute effects on birth weights, although the values observed in the non-compliant group (mean birth weight 2990 g) suggested that the effect was real. Although maternal weight increment was significantly greater in the VN group than in the PUR group (12.6 versus 11.6 kg), the observed similarity in the post partum weight was unexpected. No negative effects on fetal growth were attributed to the use of these supplements. This is not unexpected, as both supplements had an appropriate protein:energy ratio of 20% (PUR) and 12% (VN).

As previously mentioned, the effect of supplementation on birth weight has been very modest, except in very poorly nourished populations. Therefore the recent study by Doyle *et al.* (1990) is of interest, as it showed important differences in the nutrient intake in early pregnancy in women giving birth to infants less than 2500 g compared with those giving birth to infants greater than 3500 g. That there should be such differences in nutrient intake as were reported (20% less energy and protein, and 25% less folic acid in the former compared with the later group) is worthy of note. The modest effect of supplementation on birth weight is even more disappointing in the light of these data. The authors (Doyle *et al.* 1990) identified magnesium as having the greatest influence: intake was strongly correlated with birth weight and head size. There were similar correlations for iron and zinc. It is possible therefore that micronutrients, particularly minerals, may play an important part in embryonic development. The correlations between maternal nutrient intake and birth dimensions are of interest and may reflect inadequacy in some aspects of the mother's diet before conception.

Finally, it should be remembered that the benefits of any supplementation programme may become apparent in the next generation of women, for improving the health and nutritional status of infants should lay the foundation of improved reproductive performance in later life.

INTRAUTERINE NUTRITION AND INTELLECTUAL PERFORMANCE AND DISEASE PROGRAMMING FOR LATER LIFE

Some adverse effects of poor intrauterine nutrition can be offset by good postnatal care. However, there are well documented studies that show that an individual is handicapped for life either physically or mentally as a result of a poor intrauterine environment, and therefore their full genetic potential is not achieved.

Fetal malnutrition has been shown to alter normal developmental process in several species of animal. Depending on the timing of the dietary deficiency, degeneration of the cerebral cortex, the medulla and the spinal chord can be produced. Low birth weight has for some time been reported to be associated with reduced intelligence. Hill *et al.* (1984) reported the developmental outcome of 33 infants who were classed as malnourished on clinical examination, and 13 infants who were clinically well nourished. The infants came from middle to high socioeconomic groups, and were of at least 37 weeks gestation when they were born. Results indicated that at 14 years of age, children who had been malnourished had a lower IQ than their well nourished counterparts (104 ± 15 versus 121 ± 13, mean ± SD). The authors reported that the malnourished infants had a greater need for special education compared with the well nourished group. The numbers in this study are small, but do confirm results from earlier reports where larger numbers were used. Weiner *et al.* (1968) followed 417 low birth weight children and 405 full-term children from birth to 8–10 years, monitoring mental development. Differences in IQ were found between low birth weight and control children.

Valuable insights into the influence of intrauterine nutrition on the development of diet-related diseases in later life have recently emerged. In a study of 5654 men born between 1911 and 1930, it was reported that those individuals with the lowest weight at birth and at 1 year of age had the highest rate of death from ischaemic heart disease (Barker *et al.* 1989).

Fetal and placental size and the risk of hypertension in adult life were examined by Barker *et al.* (1990). The subjects (male and female), 449 in total, were born in Sharoe Green Hospital, Lancashire, between 1935 and

1943. Clinical measurements at birth, including growth data, had been recorded in unusual detail. Both systolic and diastolic blood pressure in later life were reported to be strongly related to placental weight and birth weight in both sexes. Mean systolic blood pressure increased with increasing placental weight, and decreased as birth weight increased. As the placental weight increased from less than 500 g to more than 700 g there was an increase in 1.5 mmHg in mean systolic pressure. A mean fall of 11 mmHg was recorded as birth weight rose from less than 2.5 kg to over 3.4 kg (Fig. 2.4). Other factors were associated with high blood pressure, including BMI and alcohol consumption, but the relationships between birth and placental weight and blood pressure in later life were independent of these factors. The authors concluded that the highest blood pressures occurred in men and women who had been small babies, with low birth weights and heavy placentas. The data also showed

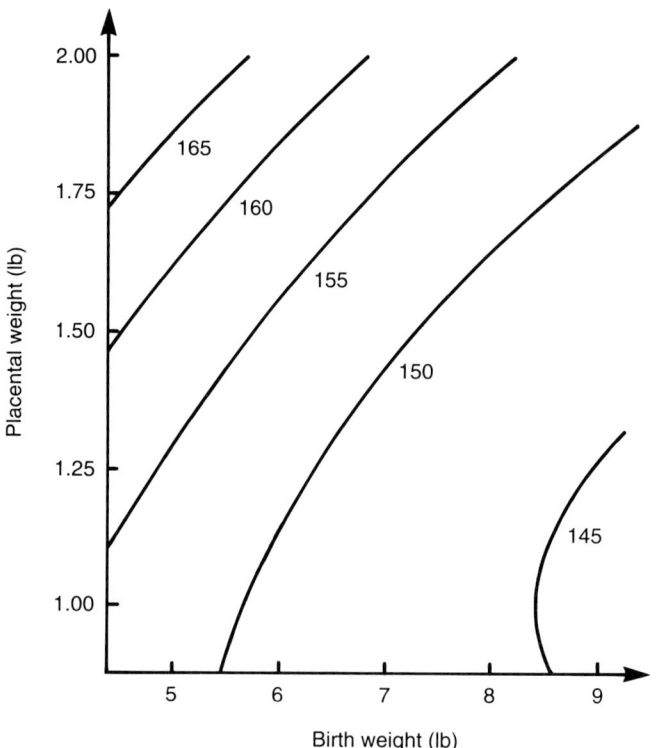

Figure 2.4 Systolic pressure (mmHg) in adult life according to placental weight and birth weight. (Reproduced with permission from Barker *et al.*, 1990.)

that the mother's external conjugate diameter (i.e. pelvic size) is strongly related to birth weight, which is consistent with existing knowledge on the relationship between maternal height and birth weight. A woman's body size depends partly on her nutritional status in childhood. There may be a link between the nutrition of young women and blood pressure in the next generation. Reducing blood pressure in a population (and thus premature deaths from cardiovascular disease and cerebrovascular accidents) may depend on improving the nutritional status of girls and women.

CONCLUSIONS

There is no doubt that a healthy well nourished woman living in comfortable surroundings is well able to provide a suitable environment for the appropriate growth of her unborn child, and is able to accumulate reserves that could protect the fetus against short periods of deprivation. However, this idealized state masks innumerable situations where a woman's lifestyle is compromised, which in turn may compromise the well-being of her baby, and the successful outcome of her pregnancy.

This chapter has highlighted aspects of the impact of maternal nutrition intake on the newborn. It is apparent that good nutritional status in a woman of reproductive age is of paramount importance in the successful outcome of pregnancy in successive generations.

REFERENCES

Barker, D.J.P., Winter, P.D., Osmond, C. *et al.* (1989) Weight in infancy and death from ischemic heart disease. *Lancet*, ii, 577–580.

Barker, D.J.P., Bull. A.R., Osmond, C. and Simmonds, S.J. (1990) Fetal and placental size and risk of hypertension in adult life. *British Medical Journal*, 301, 259–262.

Bleumink, E.C. (1983) Immunological aspects of food allergy. *Proceedings of the Nutrition Society*, 42, 219–231.

Brostoff, J. (1987) Mechanisms: an introduction. In *Food Allergy and Tolerance*, pp. 433–455 (eds J. Brostoff and S.J. Challacombe). London: Tindall.

Bruce, M.G. and Ferguson, A. (1986) Oral tolerance to ovalbumin in mice: studies of chemically modified and biologically filtered antigen. *Immunology*, 57, 627–630.

Burrell, M. and Tanner, J.M. (1961) Age at menarche in South African Bantu school girls living in the Transkei Reserve. *Human Biology*, 33, 250–261.

Cant, A.J., Bailes, J.A., Marsden, R.A. and Hewitt, D. (1986) Effect of maternal dietary exclusion on breast fed infants with eczema: two controlled studies. *British Medical Journal*, 293, 231–233.

DHSS (UK) (1979) *Recommended Daily Amounts of Food Energy and Nutrients for Groups of People in the United Kingdom*. Reports on Health and Social Subjects no. 15. London: HMSO.

Doyle, W., Crawford, M.A., Wynn, A.H.A. and Wynn, S.W. (1990) The association between maternal diet and birth dimensions. *Journal of Nutritional Medicine*, 1, 9–17.

Dreizen, S., Spirakis, C. and Stone, R. (1967) A comparison of skeletal growth and maturity in undernourished and well-nourished populations. *Journal of Pediatrics*, 70, 256–263.

Driscoll, P., Josephs, F. and Nakamoto, T. (1990) Prenatal effects of maternal caffeine intake and dietary high protein on mandibular development in fetal rats. *British Journal of Nutrition*, 63, 285–292.

Durnin, J.V.G.A. (1987) Energy requirements of pregnancy: an integration of the longitudinal data from the five-country study. *Lancet*, ii, 1131–1133.

Durnin, J.V.G.A., McKillop, F.M., Grant, S. and Fitzgerald, G. (1987) Energy requirements of pregnancy in Scotland. *Lancet*, ii, 897–900.

FAO/WHO/UNU (1985) *Energy and Protein Requirements*. WHO Technical Report Series 724. Geneva: World Health Organization.

Forsum, E., Sadurskis, A. and Wager, J. (1988) Resting metabolic rate and body composition of healthy Swedish women during pregnancy. *American Journal of Clinical Nutrition*, 47, 942–947.

Frish, R. (1978) Population, food intake and fertility. *Science*, 199, 22–30.

Furuhashi, N., Sato, S., Suzuki, M. *et al.* (1985) Effects of caffeine ingestion during pregnancy. *Gynecologic and Obstetric Investigations*, 19, 187–191.

Gant, N.F. and Worley, R.J. (1980) *Hypertension in Pregnancy: Concepts and Management*. New York: Appleton & Lange.

Graham, D. (1978) Caffeine: its identity, dietary course and biological effects. *Nutrition Reviews*, 36, 97–102.

Hediger, M.L., Scholl, T.O., Ances, I.G. *et al.* (1990) Rate and amount of weight gain during adolescent pregnancy: associations with maternal weight-for-height and birth weight. *American Journal of Clinical Nutrition*, 52, 793–799.

Hill, R.M., Verniaud, W.M., Deter, R.L. *et al.* (1984) The effect of intrauterine malnutrition on the term infant. *Acta Pediatrica Scandinavica*, 73, 482–487.

Hytten, F.E. and Chamberlain, G. (1980) *Clinical Physiology in Obstetrics*. Oxford: Blackwell.

Johnston, F. (1974) Control of age at menarche. *Human Biology*, 46, 159–171.

Kardjati, S., Kusin, J.A., Schofield, W.M. and de With, C. (1990) Energy supplementation in the last trimester of pregnancy in East Java, Indonesia: effect on maternal anthropometry. *American Journal of Clinical Nutrition*, 52, 987–994.

Little, R.E. (1977) Moderate alcohol use during pregnancy and decreased infant birth weight. *American Journal of Public Health*, 67, 1154–1156.

Lovegrove, J.A., Hampton, S.M., Morgan, J.B. and Marks, V. (1990) Effect of a milk-free diet on fetal cord blood milk antibody levels; a study of normal and atopic mothers. *Proceedings of the Nutrition Society*, 50, 9A.

Mardones-Santander, F., Rosso, P., Stekel, A. *et al.* (1988) Effect of a milk based food supplement on maternal nutritional status and fetal growth in underweight Chilean women. *American Journal of Clinical Nutrition*, 47, 413–419.

Merchant, K., Martorell, R. and Haas, J.D. (1990) Consequences for maternal nutrition of reproductive stress across consecutive pregnancies. *American Journal of Clinical Nutrition*, 52, 616–620.

Morgan, J.B. (1988) Nutrition for and during pregnancy. In *Nutrition in the Clinical Management of Disease*, 2nd edn, pp. 1–29 (eds J.W.T. Dickerson and H.A. Lee). London: Edward Arnold.

Naeye, R.L. (1981) Teenaged and pre-teenaged pregnancies: consequences of the fetal–maternal competition for nutrients. *Pediatrics*, 67, 146–150.

NRC (1989). *Recommended Dietary Allowances*, 10th edn. Washington, DC: National Academy Press.

Olsen, S. and Secher, N.S. (1990) A possible preventive effect of low-dose fish oil on early delivery and pre-eclampsia: indications from a 50-year-old controlled trial. *British Journal of Nutrition*, **64**, 599–609.

Prentice, A.M., Goldberg, G.R., Davies, H.L. *et al.* (1989) Energy sparing adaptations in human pregnancy assessed by whole body calorimetry. *British Journal of Nutrition*, **62**, 5–22.

Schofield, C., Stewart, I. and Wheeler, E. (1989) The diets of pregnant and post-pregnant women in different social groups in London and Edinburgh: calcium, iron, retinol, ascorbic acid and folic acid. *British Journal of Nutrition*, **62**, 363–377.

Scholl, T.O., Hediger, M.L. and Ances, I.G. (1990) Maternal growth during pregnancy and decreased infant birth weight. *American Journal of Clinical Nutrition*, **51**, 790–793.

Schorah, C.J. and Smithells, R.W. (1991) Maternal nutrition and malformations of the neural tube. *Nutrition Research Reviews*, **4**, 33–50.

Smith, C.A. (1947) Effects of maternal undernutrition upon the newborn infant in Holland. *Journal of Pediatrics*, **30**, 229–234.

Stevens-Simon, C. and McAnarney, E.R. (1988) Adolescent material weight gain and low birth weight: a multifactorial model. *American Journal of Clinical Nutrition*, **47**, 948–953.

Susser, M. (1981) Prenatal nutrition, birth weight, and psychological development: an overview of experiments, quasiexperiments and natural experiments in the past decade. *American Journal of Clinical Nutrition*, **34**, 784–803.

Weiner, G., Rider, R.V., Oppel, W.C. and Harper, P.A. (1968) Correlates of low birth weight psychological status at 8 to 10 years of age. *Pediatric Research*, **2**, 110–118.

Whitelaw, A. (1991) The newborn baby. In *Child Health*, 2nd edn, pp. 95–106 (eds D. Harrey and I. Kovar). Edinburgh: Churchill Livingstone.

Worthington-Roberts, B.S., Vermeersch, J. and Rodwell Williams, S. (1985) *Nutrition in Pregnancy and Lactation*, 3rd edn. St Louis, MO: Times Mirror/Mosby College Publishing.

Wright, J. (1988) Nutrition and alcohol. In *Nutrition in the Clinical Management of Disease*, 2nd edn, pp. 440–455 (eds J.W.T. Dickerson and H.A. Lee). London: Edward Arnold.

Wynn, A. (1987) Nutrition before conception and the outcome of pregnancy. *Nutrition and Health*, **5**, 31–43.

3
Patterns and determinants of infant feeding practices worldwide

Jean King
Cancer Research Campaign, London, UK
Ann Ashworth
Centre for Human Nutrition, London School of Hygiene and Tropical Medicine, London, UK

INTRODUCTION

The many advantages of breast milk over other foods for early infant feeding and the hazards of artificial milks and bottle feeding, especially in the context of developing countries, are now well established and have been described in detail elsewhere (Hanson, 1988; Jelliffe and Jelliffe, 1988). For nutritional, immunological, contraceptive, psychological and economic reasons, breast feeding remains superior. Although the impact of breast feeding on infectious disease rates in Western industrialized countries has been questioned (Bauchner *et al.* 1986), the weight of evidence remains in favour of a protective role, especially against diarrhoeal and respiratory diseases and some allergic conditions. In Third World countries, beset by poverty and adverse living conditions, breast feeding is vital for infant health. Since access to modern contraceptive methods may also be limited, breast feeding plays a major role in child spacing. This in turn benefits maternal and child health, and indirectly benefits the national economy. Conversely, the purchase of imported infant milk products has a negative economic impact at both the household and national level.

Despite the many benefits of breast feeding, a decline in its practice has been observed worldwide. In this chapter we begin by describing recent trends and current infant feeding practices in a number of countries. We then discuss some of the likely reasons for these practices, highlighting their varying impact under different circumstances, and we look at some

Infant Nutrition. Edited by A.F. Walker and B.A. Rolls.
Published in 1994 by Chapman & Hall, London.
ISBN 0 412 59140 5.

recent breast feeding promotion programmes. Finally, using these data, we consider measures that are likely to be most effective in promoting breast feeding.

CONTEMPORARY PATTERNS OF INFANT FEEDING

Caution must be exercised when comparing studies of infant feeding practices both within and between cultures, as a number of weaknesses in method are often found which are likely to bias the results. For example, studies may be restricted to a particular ecological region, socioeconomic or ethnic subgroup, and frequently the sample is based on clinic or hospital attendees. Investigators may also fail to control for confounding factors and a number of terms relating to infant feeding are used rather loosely in the literature, leading to confusion and misinterpretation: the definitions for several key terms used in this chapter are listed in Table 3.1

Infant feeding practices in Western countries

Initiation and duration of breast feeding

A decline in the duration of breast feeding was observed concurrently with industrialization and urbanization, and was associated with the increased employment of women. Thus lactation commonly lasted only 7 months in the UK during the 19th century, which also saw the development of the glass feeding bottle and the rubber teat, and the first marketing of processed milks: by 1883 27 brands of proprietary infant foods were available. This was the beginning of the era of 'scientific' infant feeding, characterized by a regimented feeding schedule and a shift in authority away from female midwives and towards male doctors (King and Ashworth, 1987). Both initiation and duration of breast feeding continued to decline throughout the first seven decades of the 20th century so that by 1975 only 51% of mothers in England and Wales initiated breast feeding and only 9% continued for 6 months (Martin, 1978).

A similar decline in the initiation and duration of breast feeding was observed in the USA. Then, in the early 1980s, a reversal in the downward trend began, which was mirrored in the UK. In large, nationwide studies, the proportion of mothers who initiated breast feeding rose to about 60% and over one-quarter were still breast feeding at 5–6 months. There is now evidence, however, that, in the UK and USA at least, this upward trend has either reached a plateau, or may in fact be in reverse (Table 3.2).

Indeed, the US data, which were derived from questionnaires mailed to large samples of mothers representative of the national distribution of

Table 3.1 Definitions used in this chapter

Term	Definition
Exclusive breast feeding	Breast feeding with or without supplements of water, fruit juice or vitamins
Supplementation	Use of other milk and/or other foods together with breast milk
Sevrage	Total replacement of breast milk with other milk and/or other food
Other milk	Processed milk or fresh animal milk. Processed milk specified where known as infant formula, sweetened condensed milk or dried milk powder
Terms avoided	*Reason*
Weaning	Used by some to indicate termination of breast feeding and by others the introduction of supplementary foods
Bottle feeding	Does not specify what is being given in the bottle
Mixed feeding	Does not specify whether breast milk is being given
Other terms used	
Western countries	Denotes industrialized countries, e.g. Europe, USA, Australia
Third World countries	Used for brevity: denotes technologically developing countries

births, have been criticized on the grounds that they may overestimate the actual prevalence of breast feeding. For, in spite of adjusting for income, education and ethnicity to reflect census data, the reported figures remain higher than in several other studies. It is suggested that non-respondents (almost half in 1984) are more likely to lack permanent mailing addresses, to be of lower socioeconomic status and have lower rates of breast feeding than respondents, and that failure to control adequately for the difference in response rates has biased the results (Rassin *et al.* 1984). In the UK, national data have been derived from questionnaires mailed to samples of mothers drawn from the census lists. The response rate has been better

Table 3.2 Trends in breast feeding practices in three Western regions: percentages of mothers breast feeding for different periods

	Ever	3–4 months	5–6 months	9 months	References
1950s					
USA	<29				a
UK (1959–1965)	31–83	5–29	13		b(i)
1970s					
USA (1971)	25	8	5		a
UK (1975)	51	13	9		b(ii)
W. Australia (1972)	<50				c
Early 1980s					
USA (1982)	62	38	29		a
UK (1980)	65	26	22	12	b(iii)
W. Australia (1980)	82				c
Late 1980s					
USA (1984)	60	35	26		a
USA (1987)	55				a
UK (1985)	64	26	21	11	b(iii)
W. Australia (1985)	86	62	45	28	c

[a] USA data from Martinez and Krieger (1985) and Ryan and Martinez (1989).
[b] UK data from (i), Oppé (1974), (ii), Martin and Monk (1982), (iii) Martin and White (1988).
[c] Australia data taken from Hitchcock and Coy (1988).

than in the USA: in 1985, 91%, 73% and 61% of mothers responded at 6 weeks, 4 months and 9 months respectively after the birth of their babies (Martin and White, 1988).

In some Western countries, however, it appears that the return to breast feeding has not only been maintained but has continued to increase. Thus in Western Australia and Tasmania a survey in 1984–1985 found that over 80% of mothers were breast feeding on discharge from hospital, and 45% were still breast feeding at 6 months. Breast milk was the only source of milk given by over three-quarters of mothers on discharge and by over half at 3 months. This survey was one of a series dating back to the 1950s in which a continuous decline in breast feeding had been observed, reaching a nadir around 1970, when fewer than half of Western Australian mothers breast fed on leaving hospital. By the late 1970s the proportion had risen to over 80%. Local factors associated with this dramatic increase are considered later but it is noteworthy that the resurgence was first seen among the higher socioeconomic groups, and breast feeding remains more prevalent and sustained in these groups (Hitchcock and Coy, 1988). High rates of breast feeding are also reported for the Netherlands and Canada

(Lawrence and Friedman, 1990) and for Scandinavia (Kocturk and Zetterstrom, 1989; WHO, 1989a).

Supplementation patterns

In 19th-century Britain, supplements of bread, pap or a 'panada' of cereals cooked in broth were given in the first week of life (King and Ashworth, 1987). In line with a worldwide trend among industrialized countries, the nature of the first supplement has changed from a traditional pap to various types of processed milk, to the almost universal use of infant formulas. In the USA, the shift away from evaporated and cows' milk to formula was complete by the mid-1960s (Martinez and Krieger, 1985). In England and Wales in 1985, 36% of mothers gave infant formula feeds from birth, and by 6 weeks of age the majority of infants were being fed on infant formula with or without breast feeds: the proportion of breast-fed infants receiving formula supplements at 6 weeks of age rose from 66% to 72% between 1980 and 1985, indicating a trend towards earlier use of formula. Thus, exclusive breast feeding remains a rare event even in the early weeks of life. By 4 months, three-quarters of all infants were being fully bottle fed with formula (Martin and White, 1988).

In England and Wales, between 1975 and 1980, a sharp decrease in the proportion of mothers introducing solids before 3 months was observed, from 85% to 56% (62% in 1985). Non-breast-feeding mothers, smokers and those from lower social classes tend to introduce solids earlier. Cereals and rusks continue to be the commonest first solids and 90% of infants in 1985 were receiving commercial non-milk baby foods at 4 months (Martin and White, 1988). In Western Australia, few infants are introduced to solid and non-milk foods under 3 months of age: these are generally introduced at 3–4 months, starting with cereals, then fruit, desserts and vegetables. As in the UK, infants receiving artificial milks are introduced to solids earlier than breast-fed infants (Hitchcock and Coy, 1988).

Infant feeding practices in Third World countries

Initiation and duration of breast feeding

The extensive body of literature on infant feeding practices in seven technologically developing countries has recently been reviewed: Malaysia, Kenya, Nigeria, Zaire, the English-speaking Caribbean, India and Mexico. In all seven almost universal initiation of breast feeding is still found (King and Ashworth, 1991).

Typical findings for breast feeding practices in the late 1970s based on large-scale, nationally representative samples are presented in Table 3.3.

Table 3.3 Breast feeding patterns in seven developing countries in the late 1970s: results of national large-scale studies. Percentages of mothers breast feeding for different periods

Country	Ever	5–6 months	10–12 months	References
Malyasia				
Urban élite	68	11	4	
Urban poor	75	30	24	} a
Rural	85	65	44	
Caribbean				
Urban		42	18	b
Rural	>92	66	31	c
Mexico				
Urban élite	80	17	6	
Urban poor	85	45	27	} a
Rural	91	53	38	
Nigeria				
Urban élite	100	32	0	
Urban poor	100	97	97	} d
Rural	100	100	97	
Kenya				
Urban élite	98	79	54	
Urban poor	98	85	80	} a
Rural	100	99	86	
Zaire				
Urban élite	100	100	80	
Urban poor	100	100	84	} d
Rural	100	100	96	
India				
Urban élite	96	49	33	
Urban poor	99	88	93	} d
Rural	100	100	99	

Reference	Date of study	Sample size
[a]Dimond and Ashworth (1987)	1979	Over 6000 (all three countries combined)
[b]Ferry (1981)	1975–6	1973
[c]Gussler and Mock (1983)	1979	520
[d]WHO (1981)	1975–8	Over 6300 (all three countries combined)

Two distinct patterns emerge. In one, universal and prolonged lactation persists among the majority of the population. This is the case for Nigeria, Kenya, Zaire and India. In Nairobi, for example, 85% and 50% of mothers still breast feed at 6 and 15 months respectively. In all but Zaire, however, the urban élite are set apart by their shorter lactation period.

Thus in Nigeria, lactation continues up to 1 year nationally and even longer in rural areas, while among the urban élite and middle classes duration has declined and in one major study only one-third of such mothers were still breast feeding at 6 months. Similarly, in India, although prolonged lactation is the rule, half the urban élite mothers in one major study were found to stop breast feeding by 1 year. In Zaire, by contrast, nearly all mothers breast feed for at least 12 months (King and Ashworth, 1991).

The second pattern is characterized by a high initiation but decreased duration of breast feeding among the majority of mothers, with a more marked decline in urban areas. This is seen in Malaysia, the Caribbean and Mexico. Thus, while at least half of rural Malay infants are breast-fed for 6 months, fewer than one-third of urban infants are breast-fed for this period (Dimond and Ashworth, 1987). In the Caribbean, studies indicate that fewer than half of urban infants are breast-fed for 6 months compared with almost two-thirds of rural infants (Popkin *et al.* 1982). In Mexico, fewer than 10% of urban élite mothers now breast feed beyond 6 months, and only one-quarter breast feed for 3 months. Among urban poor and rural mothers, however, approximately half breast feed for up to 6 months and between one-quarter and two-fifths continue for 12 months (Dimond and Ashworth, 1987).

Clearly the circumstances that have led these mothers to stop breast feeding earlier than was previously the norm for their culture have not prevented them from breast feeding for at least a brief period. Indeed there are signs of a return to breast feeding in some Third World countries. In some, such as Brazil, Honduras, Indonesia and the Philippines, this trend is associated with national breast feeding promotion programmes which are discussed in the penultimate section of this chapter. In others, although no support programmes may have been pursued on a national level, an increased awareness within the health sector, leading to changes in health care practices that are more conducive to successful lactation, may have influenced mothers' infant feeding behaviour. Thus, in Malaysia, data from the Malaysian Family Life Survey, examined separately for each year in the 1970s, indicate that, following an all-time low reached early in the decade, rates of initiation of breast feeding had increased among all socioeconomic and ethnic groups by the late 1970s. The increase was greatest among the poorer Indian and Chinese subgroups and among women either with more than primary education or those with no education at all. It was also greater among women delivering in hospital or private maternity clinics. In the early 1970s only 20% of such infants were breast-fed, compared with 93% of infants born at home, but this difference appears to have narrowed considerably for infants born in 1975–1977. Among infants born to poor Chinese or Indian families, 51% of hospital- or clinic-born infants were breast-fed in 1970–1974, increasing to 70% in 1975–1977. The increased prevalence is believed to indicate successful implementation of measures within the health sector to promote and support breast feeding (Haaga, 1986). In Indonesia too, an increase in breast feeding rates has been observed among mothers from lower socioeconomic groups (Joesoef *et al.* 1989), in contrast to the experience in Western countries where it is mothers from higher social groups who have led the breast feeding revival.

Supplementation patterns

Until recently, it was assumed that, in pre-industrial societies, all mothers breast fed exclusively for several months. It is now recognized, however, that in a wide range of cultures mothers have traditionally provided supplements to their infants from an early age (King and Ashworth, 1987). Three main factors appear to be involved. First, in many cultures colostrum has been rejected and substituted with pre-lacteal feeds. Second, there has existed a widespread cultural perception of the nourishing or 'superfood' qualities of the local staple, coupled with the belief that breast milk alone is an inadequate food. Third, in many societies the women's agricultural or other work commitment has required that the infant be left for perhaps several hours at a time with a caretaker, when some alternative to breast milk must be provided (Carballo and Pelto, 1991).

In those societies where early supplements were traditionally given, this practice has persisted into modern times, but often the nature of the supplements has changed, as shown in Table 3.4. Moreover, in many cultures where supplementation was traditionally begun later there has been a trend towards earlier introduction of other foods, for example in Nigeria, Mexico and urban India. Whereas the traditional first supplement offered to infants around the world was usually a gruel prepared from the local staple, this has now largely been replaced in the first semester by infant formula and commercial cereals, reflecting the trend observed in Western countries. Of the seven countries surveyed, the traditional first food has continued to be used by the majority in only two: Zaire and rural India. By the second semester, however, only in Mexico and the Caribbean are the commercial supplements continued: in the other five countries, the traditional gruel reasserts itself in the older infant's diet (King and Ashworth, 1991).

Summary of contemporary infant feeding practices

In 1982, the World Health Organization defined three basic 'phases' in breast feeding prevalence and duration: phase 1 was the 'traditional phase' with both high prevalence and duration; phase 2 was the so-called 'transformation phase' with prevalence falling and duration becoming

Table 3.4 Traditional and contemporary patterns of supplementation

Country	Timing of supplementation	Nature of main supplement	
		First semester	*Second semester*
Malaysia			
Traditional	Early	Banana/rice gruel	Gruel contd[a]
Contemporary	Early	IF, commercial cereal[b]	Traditional gruel [a,c]
Kenya			
Traditional	Early	Cows' milk/maize gruel	Thicker gruel[a]
Contemporary	Early	Processed milk including IF, some commercial cereal[b]	Traditional gruel[a]
Nigeria			
Traditional	Medium–late	Maize or sorghum gruel	Gruel contd[a]
Contemporary	Early	IF (declining?)[b]	Traditional gruel[c]
Zaire			
Traditional	Early–medium	Traditional gruel	Gruel contd[a]
Contemporary	Early–medium	Traditional gruel (Limited IF in urban areas)	Gruel contd[a]
Caribbean			
Traditional	Early–late	Cereal/starchy gruel	Gruel contd[a]
Contemporary	Early	IF, commercial cereal	Traditional gruel Processed milk[a,d]
India			
Traditional	Late	Animal milk	Animal milk
Contemporary	Late, rural Early–medium urban	IF, animal milk commercial cereal[b]	Animal milk[a]
Mexico			
Traditional	Late	Animal milk, soup-soaked cornbread, maize gruel	Gruel contd[a]
Contemporary	Early	IF	Commercial cereals

Source: King and Ashworth (1991).
IF, infant formula.
Timing defined as commonly given: early, <3 months; medium, 3–6 months; late >6 months. Supplementation defined as excluding pre-lacteal and early feeding of infusions and teas.
[a]Including gradual progression to an adult-type diet.
[b]Predominantly in urban areas, to a lesser extent in rural areas.
[c]Elite mothers continue use of infant formula and commercial cereals.
[d]Reversal of decline towards prolonged breast feeding by élite mothers.

shorter; and phase 3 was the 'resurgence phase' with rising prevalence and duration (WHO, 1982). Within any country or region different segments of the population might be in a different phase. Thus, in many developing countries, while the higher socioeconomic group was predominantly in phase 2, the rest of the population remained in phase 1. Conversely, in many Western countries, the higher socioeconomic groups were in phase 3 and the rest were in phase 2. In other words, a shift was observed away from breast feeding by élite Third World mothers at the same time that élite Western mothers were returning to it.

We have found, however, that the three-phase model does not adequately describe current patterns of breast feeding: in many Third World countries a high initial rate of breast feeding remains, but this is of short duration and, even where duration is long, this may be combined with very early supplementation (Popkin *et al.* 1982; King and Ashworth, 1991; Winikoff and Laukaran, 1989). Moreover, in some Western countries, the resurgence observed in the late 1970s and early 1980s appears to have been partial or temporary (e.g. Martin and White, 1988). In others, however, as we have seen, there is a sustained rise both in initiation and duration of breast feeding. In addition, in some Third World countries where efforts have been made to promote and support breast feeding, there are indications of a return to longer periods of lactation. Thus, there are at least five rather than three phases which can be described, as shown in Table 3.5.

The observation of various breast feeding 'phases' has resulted in the 'cultural diffusion' theory which sees the behaviour of the urban middle and poor classes and the rural poor as imitative of the urban élite. The latter are thus considered the trend-setters in social and health behaviour. An alternative theory supposes that changes in infant feeding practices have become necessary owing to socioeconomic changes, including increased entry of women into the modern labour market, the breakdown of traditional support networks and the general pressures of modern urban lifestyles (WHO, 1982). We shall now consider the evidence for these explanations of infant feeding behaviour as well as for other possible determinants of the practices described above.

DETERMINANTS OF INFANT FEEDING PRACTICES

If mothers are to be encouraged to choose to breast feed their infants and are to be supported in this choice, then an understanding of the social, cultural and economic contexts in which that choice has to be made is essential. From the literature a number of factors emerge that appear to play a greater or lesser role in influencing this decision in different parts of the world.

Table 3.5 Phases in breast feeding practices around the world

Phase	Breast feeding initiation	Breast feeding duration	Social groups	Examples
1. Traditional	High	High	All	Zaire
			Poor/rural	India, Nigeria Kenya
2. Transformation				
– partial	High	Falling	Élite	Indonesia, India Nigeria, Kenya Malaysia (Indians)
			All	Malaysia (Malays) Mexico Caribbean
3. Transformation				
– severe	Low	Falling	Élite	Malaysia (Chinese)
4. Resurgence	Risen	Risen		
– partial	Static/falling	Static/falling	All	UK, USA
5. Resurgence				
– active	Rising	Rising	All, led by élite	Australia, Scandinavia Brazil, Honduras, Philippines
	High	Rising	Poor	Indonesia
	Rising	?	Poor	Malaysia (Indians, Chinese)

Maternal characteristics associated with breast feeding in Western countries

In the studies from England and Wales and the USA, reported above, a number of factors have been shown to be associated with the initiation and/or duration of breast feeding and these are summarized in Table 3.6.

In all three national surveys in England and Wales, the highest rates of breast feeding initiation were found among mothers of first babies (particularly if their first baby was born when they were over 25 years of age), those in higher social classes, educated beyond the age of 18, and living in

Table 3.6 Maternal and sociocultural characteristics and health practices associated with low rates of breast feeding (initiation and/or duration) in US and UK studies: targets for intervention

(a)	*Maternal sociocultural characteristics*
	Young age
	Short period of education
	Low income/social class
	Smoker
	Single mother (UK)
	Black mother (USA)
	Complicated delivery
	No previous breast feeding experience
	Early return to full-time work (USA)
(b)	*Health sector practices*
	Delay in first putting infant to breast
	Separation of mother and infant
	Scheduled feeds
	Routine supplementation
	Free gift of infant formula

south-east England. The longer a mother had breast fed a first baby, the more likely she was to breast feed again, and mothers who smoked were less likely to start breast feeding than non-smokers. In the 1980 and 1985 studies, there was no evidence that mothers who were working outside the home 6 weeks after the birth of their babies were less likely to have initiated breast feeding than non-working mothers. Each of the above factors was independently associated with the initiation of breast feeding.

Factors found to be associated with continuing to breast feed for at least 6 weeks included previous experience of breast feeding, higher social class, education beyond 18 years of age, residence in the south of England, and being a non-smoker. In 1985, no evidence was found that returning to work significantly shortened breast feeding duration (although in the earlier studies this was the case) (Martin and White, 1988).

In the USA, higher rates of initiation and duration of breast feeding have similarly been found to be associated with maternal age, longer duration of education and higher socioeconomic status, with non-smoking and previous successful breast feeding (Feinstein *et al.* 1986; Martinez and Krieger, 1985). In addition, several studies have shown a strong association with ethnic group, lower rates of breast feeding being found among black compared with Anglo-American mothers (Rassin *et al.* 1984; Lawrence and Friedman, 1990). The national data for 1987 indicate that, while full-time employment outside the home does not influence overall rates of breast feeding initiation, only half as many working mothers still breast feed by 6 months (Ryan and Martinez, 1989). The influence of employment on infant feeding practices is discussed in more detail below.

Maternal characteristics associated with breast feeding in Third World countries

In contrast to Western countries, breast feeding in Third World countries is associated with lower income and social class, and with rural living. The greatest decline in breast feeding has been seen among urban élite mothers (Table 3.3), who have higher levels of education and are more likely to be employed in the modern sector. In some societies, feeding with infant formula has become associated with being modern and progressive, while breast feeding has acquired a 'primitive' and 'backward' image (King and Ashworth, 1987).

Women's work roles: the experience in Western countries

Recent evidence in the UK indicates that neither the initiation nor the length of breast feeding is influenced by full-time work outside the home. In the USA there is some evidence of a negative impact, particularly on duration (Kurinij *et al.* 1989). The time at which work is resumed may be important. For example, in the USA, mothers who returned to work more than 16 weeks after giving birth, and those who worked part-time, were found to breast feed for longer than other working mothers (Auerbach and Guss, 1984), and black women planning to work part-time were more likely to initiate breast feeding compared with those planning to work full-time (controlling for other variables). Mothers in professional occupations had a longer duration of breast feeding than those returning to non-professional work (Kurinij *et al.* 1989).

It is clear therefore that breast feeding is not intrinsically incompatible with women's employment, but it is an activity that must compete with multiple pressures from other economic and domestic roles (Lawrence and Friedman, 1990). One reason why working mothers may breast feed for shorter periods, particularly if full-time or non-professional, is that a lower frequency of suckling may, coupled with fatigue, result in reduced milk output (Ryan and Martinez, 1989). This in turn may fuel maternal concerns over 'insufficient milk' (discussed below), leading to anxiety, which may further inhibit the 'let-down' reflex. Fewer suckling episodes may also lead to breast problems such as engorgement: these might be avoided by increased breast feeding at night and by the use of breast pumps during the day to empty the breasts.

Women's work roles: the Third World experience

In the comparative study of changes in infant feeding patterns in seven developing countries described above, it is noteworthy that a departure from traditional practices was first observed in the Caribbean and Malaysia, where a large proportion of women worked in the commercial agricultural sector. This necessitated long periods of separation from their infants, and the trend towards use of processed milks began early in the 20th century, replacing the traditional gruels that had previously been used as breast milk supplements and substitutes. Women still comprise 40% of the workforce in Malaysia, while 30% of households in the Caribbean are headed by women (King and Ashworth, 1987). Similarly, in Mexico, women's paid employment is associated with a shorter duration of lactation, and in one study one-third of working mothers had not breast fed at all (Cardenas *et al.* 1981).

Even in more traditional societies, women's work roles may be incompatible with exclusive breast feeding, and supplements are often provided at an early age while the mother is working in the fields (Carballo and Pelto, 1991). This is the case in some parts of Zaire where, it has been suggested, poor maternal nutritional status may result in the mother being unable to fulfil all the energy-consuming activities expected of her. Even where nutritional status is not a constraint, a mother has to choose between the many conflicting demands on her time and may decide that it is more cost-effective to substitute another member of the household in the infant feeding role (Butz, 1977). In both Nigeria and Kenya, however, as in some parts of Zaire, traditional work roles do not appear to conflict with breast feeding (King and Ashworth, 1987).

Similarly, in a review of 16 Third World studies comparing infant feeding practices among non-working and working mothers, eight reported no significant difference between the two groups, four found a negative and four a mixed relationship between mothers' work and breast feeding. Allowing for various method weaknesses, the author concludes that this lack of a definite pattern is consistent with other studies in which women have been asked their reason for not initiating breast feeding or for terminating breast feeding early. In most, very few women gave work as a reason. In a similar analysis of 10 studies which compared the nutritional status of children of working versus non-working mothers, inconsistent results were again found. The author suggests that, in some contexts, the negative effect of reduced breast feeding may be offset by the positive economic effects of maternal employment (Leslie, 1985).

Maternal attitudes and beliefs: the Western experience

In many studies from around the world, maternal decisions on infant feeding have been shown to be based, either wholly or in part, on a consideration of optimal health for the mother or her child. This might be reflected in concern over insufficient milk, medical problems, or opinions regarding the relative merits of breast milk versus infant formula (Carballo and Pelto, 1991). Such concerns can lead to either breast or formula feeding being chosen, especially where certain types of maternal behaviour, such as smoking and consuming non-nutritious foods, are viewed as potentially harmful: in these circumstances mothers may prefer not to breast feed (Gabriel *et al.* 1986).

In the national studies in England and Wales, the main reasons given for breast feeding were a perception by the mother that breast milk was best for the baby and that it was more convenient (Martin and Monk, 1982; Martin and White, 1988). Other reasons commonly given were that breast feeding was natural and facilitated mother–infant bonding, that it was cheaper and, for mothers with more than one child, because of a favourable earlier lactation experience. The main reasons given for formula feeding were that others could feed the baby, previous unfavourable experience of breast feeding, and embarrassment or dislike of breast feeding. The most frequently given reason for stopping breast feeding at all ages was a perceived insufficiency of milk. Sore nipples and other breast problems were the next most common reason for stopping within 2 weeks, while at a later age the time taken to breast feed was the next reason cited and, for sevrage after 4 months, that the mother had breast fed for as long as intended (Martin and White, 1988).

Maternal attitudes and beliefs: the Third World experience

As noted above, in many traditional societies breast milk was not always considered to be in itself a sufficient food, whereas great faith was placed in the local staple. This faith has, to some extent, been transferred to commercial products and mothers may use them as a tonic or nutrient booster to breast milk. Nevertheless, the high prevalence of breast feeding is evidence that the majority of Third World mothers still recognize the health and nutritional value of breast milk (Winikoff and Laukaran, 1989). In some countries, such as Nigeria and Zaire, an increase in 'modern' monogamous marriages in urban areas, coupled with retention of the traditional taboo on sexual intercourse during lactation, has resulted in a shortening of the breast feeding period. There may also exist a desire to emulate the élite, who use infant formula more frequently, while some reports have noted a perception of breast feeding as 'primitive' (King and Ashworth, 1987).

The 'insufficient milk' syndrome

Around the world, the most common reason cited either for not breast feeding at all or for early cessation is a perceived insufficient supply of breast milk (e.g. King and Ashworth, 1987; Winikoff and Laukaran, 1989). While in the Third World context there may sometimes be a genuine deficit in milk production due to poor maternal nutritional status and an onerous workload, it is likely that in most cases this perceived insufficiency is related to inadequate suckling. It is often the infant's behaviour, such as crying and restlessness, that generates this belief and leads to maternal insecurity and anxiety, which may in turn adversely affect the 'let-down' reflex. Feeding on demand, which has been the traditional form of breast feeding through the ages, may reflect a physiological need designed to provide sufficient stimulus for milk synthesis (Carballo and Pelto, 1991). What is clear is that the response of many mothers, who in the Western or urban setting are often unable to spare the time for prolonged demand feeding, is to supplement their perceived inadequate supply of milk with bottle feeds of infant formula. If insufficient suckling is causing the low milk supply, this response will only compound the problem. However, there are other reasons why infants are fretful, such as colic, and mothers need to be made aware both of the need to increase the frequency of suckling and to investigate alternative causes of infant distress.

Influences on maternal attitudes

Numerous studies have addressed the role of individuals or networks in providing informal support to the breast feeding mother. In many traditional societies an older woman, the *doula*, fulfils this role while in others the presence of the extended family means that experienced advice is always to hand. With urbanization this traditional support has often been lost. For example, in the USA, the mother's mother is no longer the main advisor, being replaced by a male partner (white mothers) or close friend (black and Hispanic mothers) (Bryant, 1982; Carballo and Pelto, 1991). Clearly it is important to take account of these sources of influence when developing breast feeding promotional strategies.

The commercial promotion of infant formula

The commercial promotion of processed milks as substitutes for breast milk began in the second half of the 19th century in Western countries and as early as the 1920s in some Third World countries with a large expatriate population, such as Malaysia. Increasingly, advertisements for infant foods were directed towards the local population, and by the 1950s advertisements appeared regularly in local newspapers in Malaysia and the Caribbean. In Nigeria, however, it was not until the 1960s that wide-spread promotion of processed milk for infants occurred and, by the late 1970s, there were over 40 brands of milk and milk-based products and 11 brands of feeding bottle on the market, and an estimated 1% of total sales volume was given free, mainly to private health institutions (WHO, 1981).

In Zaire, by contrast, there has been little commercial promotion of infant foods. This may be related to Zaire's very low GNP, which places it amongst the poorest nations of the world and consequently reduces its commercial attractiveness to international companies. Since 1981, when the WHO Code of Marketing of Breast-milk Substitutes was passed by the Assembly of the World Health Organization, only a few countries, including Kenya and Mexico, have ratified the Code but over 70, including Zaire, Nigeria, Malaysia, India and some Caribbean countries, are awaiting legislation or have partly enacted the Code. These have prohibit-ed the advertising of infant formula in the mass media and direct contact of company personnel with mothers. There has, however, been an enor-mous upsurge in the advertising of 'follow-on' milks, and hospitals contin-ue to request and accept excessive quantities of infant formula, donated by companies (Palmer, 1988).

Although some countries have adopted the WHO Code on a voluntary, less forceful basis, or have produced a weaker version, others have taken a very firm stand: in Papua New Guinea for example, feeding bottles may only be obtained on prescription. In addition, the serious socioeconomic setbacks due to the world recession of the 1980s and 1990s have led to a decline in imports of infant formula and other processed milks in some countries, which has probably had a positive impact on breast feeding rates. The importance of the commercial promotion of infant formula and its tacit endorsement via the health sector has been substantiated by stud-ies indicating the mothers' awareness of brand names and a commonly reported belief that formula is good for infants, having properties similar to 'tonic' foods (King and Ashworth, 1987; Winikoff and Laukaran, 1989).

The role of the health sector: the Western experience

A substantial body of contemporary research has addressed how hospital practices and the attitudes of health professionals have influenced infant feeding decisions.

Hospital practices in the neonatal period

A number of health sector practices which have been the routine for decades throughout the world have been shown to have a negative impact on successful lactation: these are listed in Table 3.6. In the series of national studies in England and Wales, events occurring during labour and delivery and the period immediately after the birth have been shown to be strongly associated with the successful establishment of lactation (Martin and White, 1988). Three-quarters of the 19% of mothers who stopped breast feeding in the first 2 weeks after birth did so while in hospital. Having a Caesarian delivery, especially under general anaesthetic, having a baby with a low birth weight or who had to go into special care for some other reason, are all associated with early cessation of breast feeding, indicating a failure of current hospital practices to provide adequate support to these mothers. Delay in putting the baby to the breast was the most important correlate: twice as many mothers (just over 30%) who first breast fed more than 12 hours after delivery had stopped within 2 weeks, compared with those who breast fed within 1 hour of delivery.

The 1985 survey in England and Wales revealed improvements in hospital practices with only 19% of breast feeding mothers reporting having to feed at set intervals, compared with 32% in 1980. Moreover, 'rooming-in' was more common in 1985 with 47% of mothers having their babies with them continuously, compared with only 17% in 1980. However, little change was reported in the proportion (almost half) of breast-fed babies receiving supplementary feeds of infant formula in the first week of life (Martin and White, 1988).

We have noted earlier how scheduled breast feeds and 'topping-up' with infant formula diminish the amount of suckling which in turn will affect the overall milk supply. In a study of US mothers who were partly breast feeding, only those who nursed at least seven times a day had breast feeding durations as long as mothers who were exclusively breast feeding. Significantly fewer of the remaining partial breast feeders continued either to 10 or 16 weeks, so that the critical factor for continued successful lactation seemed to be a high daily frequency of suckling (Feinstein *et al.* 1986).

Several studies have looked at the effect of samples of infant formula in gift packs provided to newly delivered mothers. While no effect on breast feeding success was seen in two studies, a further two found significant differences in the duration of exclusive breast feeding, with mothers who received formula having a shorter breast feeding duration. One study also showed that receiving formula had a negative impact on the length of partial breast feeding and the earlier introduction of solid foods among young, low-income mothers (who are deemed to be at greatest risk in terms of achieving prolonged breast feeding) (Frank *et al.* 1987).

Knowledge and attitudes of health workers

A survey of knowledge and attitudes related to infant feeding in one large US municipal hospital found that a substantial proportion of both clinical and nursing staff held views that were either incorrect or inconducive to the promotion of breast feeding: for example, that schedule feeds were more beneficial than feeding on demand, that infants with diarrhoea should be taken off the breast for some time, that breast feeding should be stopped in cases of sore nipples and other breast problems, that formula supplementation was beneficial, and that distribution of formula samples was appropriate (Winikoff *et al.* 1986). In order to rectify these incorrect views, an in-house training programme was developed which included educational materials for both staff and mothers. Following this programme, the incidence of breast feeding in the hospital increased. Key aspects contributing to this success were felt to be the creation of an interdisciplinary breast feeding steering committee and of an atmosphere conducive to breast feeding, with all staff, not just trained counsellors, engaged in the support programme (Winikoff *et al.* 1987).

However, in another hospital where breast feeding was strongly advocated by staff, many mothers interviewed following discharge still opted to use formula, and the brand they chose was the one used in the hospital. The authors conclude that non-verbal endorsement of infant formula products exerted a stronger influence than the counselling in support of breast feeding, and that a total change in hospital practice was required so that routines modelled breast feeding rather than formula feeding (Reiff and Essock-Vitale, 1985). Several studies have assessed the effectiveness of trained counsellors and have shown some positive impact on infant feeding practices, but further work is needed to determine the best training and content of such counselling (Frank *et al.* 1987).

An analysis in the USA of the reasons for choosing whether or not to breast feed found that most women had some biomedical knowledge of the benefits of breast feeding, but those who chose not to breast feed felt that some of their dietary and other behaviours (e.g. smoking) were barriers to breast feeding. The authors recommend that doctors enter into a dialogue with individual mothers, taking into account their demographic and cultural background (Gabriel *et al.* 1986).

The role of the health sector: the Third World experience

A review of the historical events surrounding the introduction and increasing use of artificial milks in several Third World countries showed that from the 1920s onwards the health sector has played a major role by undermining breast feeding through the promotion of regimented feeding schedules, restrictive and inappropriate hospital practices and direct encouragement to use breast milk substitutes (King and Ashworth, 1987). By the 1950s in many parts of the world, processed milks were being distributed from clinics on a large scale, thereby adding a seal of approval to their use. These programmes were initiated at a time when there was a world surplus of dried skim milk; they created a demand which later could be met only by expensive imports. By the 1960s and throughout the 1970s, maternity units frequently served as venues for distributing free formula samples to newly delivered mothers.

In a recent comparative study in urban areas of four developing countries – Thailand, Colombia, Indonesia and Kenya – negative effects of routine hospital practices similar to those described for Western countries were reported by the mothers interviewed. Rooming-in varied from 15% of all hospital births in Bogota, Colombia, to 81% in Semarang, Indonesia, and was associated with a significantly increased likelihood of prolonged lactation among mothers who were not employed (the majority) in Bogota. The provision of 'top-up' feeds was common in Nairobi, Bogota and Semarang. In Semarang, delivery attended by a doctor was associated with an increased likelihood of early bottle feeding, while in Nairobi mothers who delivered in hospital were half as likely as other mothers to continue breast feeding to 6 weeks (controlling for other variables). In Bangkok, receipt of free samples of infant formula was associated with a decreased likelihood of continuing to breast feed beyond 3 months. Brand endorsement by health professionals was also commonly reported (Winikoff and Laukaran, 1989).

The impact of health worker attitudes is probably even greater in Third World countries than in Western ones, for not only are health professionals perceived to hold important knowledge but are also more likely to represent role models of the modern 'progressive' lifestyle. A low rate of breast feeding has been reported among health workers in several Third World countries (King and Ashworth, 1987), and even where attitudes towards breast feeding are positive, knowledge may still be incomplete, resulting in incorrect advice being given to mothers. For example, in a study in Indonesian teaching hospitals, perinatal care providers, who were supportive of breast feeding, expressed concerns about the risks of infection associated with rooming-in, believed that breast feeding was inadvisable during a range of illnesses and were unaware of the benefits of early initiation of suckling (Hull *et al.* 1989).

The need for a re-examination of practices in maternity institutions is again highlighted in a Jamaican study comparing a large urban hospital, where extensive education was provided to mothers, with a rural hospital where very little education was given. It was found that breast feeding practices in the rural centre more closely approximated recommendations and that maternal knowledge of breast feeding was no less than in the urban centre. Practices in the urban hospital, particularly delays in initiating breast feeding, lack of continuity of staff between delivery and post partum care, as well as a lack of clarification of their respective roles in relation to breast feeding support, were believed to contribute to the poor breast feeding achievement in the urban hospital and the authors conclude that educational initiatives alone are unlikely to prove effective unless accompanied by specific health practices that support breast feeding (Cunningham and Segree, 1990).

In a number of countries, institution-based measures have been taken to curtail detrimental health sector activities and implement supportive practices. A summary of some of these institutional programmes, listing their key features, is given in Table 3.7. The main focus has been on ensuring early and frequent suckling, encouragement and informed advice and avoidance of formula endorsement. Another important aspect has been the training of health personnel, not only to understand the benefits of breast feeding and the need to alter unsupportive routines, but also to recognize how few contraindications to breast feeding actually exist. An outcome of many of the programmes is that infants who would previously have been automatically put onto formula feeds are now successfully breast-fed or fed with expressed human milk. The anticipated cumulative effect over time of the various measures implemented is a shift in ethos away from routines centred around formula feeding and towards a relaxed atmosphere where breast feeding is the norm. Many of the programmes have been evaluated, with varying degrees of rigour, and the general finding is an increase in the duration of breast feeding following implementation. In hospitals in the Philippines and Costa Rica, an associated decrease in morbidity and mortality, particularly in relation to diarrhoeal diseases, has also been observed (Jelliffe and Jelliffe, 1988).

NATIONAL PROGRAMMES TO PROMOTE AND PROTECT BREAST FEEDING

In addition to the institution-based programmes described above, a number of countries have, since the mid-1970s, launched national programmes to promote breast feeding. Four examples are given in Table 3.8 to illustrate their main features. Besides those countries listed, national programmes have also been initiated in Canada, Colombia, Jamaica, Papua New Guinea and Thailand. Crucial to the success of such programmes is the involvement and commitment of all relevant ministries and agencies in a coordinated multidisciplinary approach.

All the programmes have focused on educational activities, targeting in particular the health sector and mothers. Increasingly too, emphasis is

Table 3.7 Key features of some institutional programmes to promote breast feeding

Features	Finland	Italy	Philippines	India	Costa Rica
1. Mother–infant contact/breast feeding initiation within 3h of delivery	+	+	+	+	+
2. Rooming-in	+		+	+	+
3. Breast feeding on demand	+		+	+	
4. Breast feeding encouraged for difficult deliveries (e.g. Caesarians)		+	+[a]		
5. Breast milk/colostrum given to pre-term and high-risk neonates			+[a]	+[a]	+
6. Supplementation restricted/banned	+	+	+	+	
7. Human milk banks established			+	+	+
8. Seminars/involvement of staff	+	+	+	+	+
9. Information/counselling to mother	+		+	+	+
10. Post-discharge support (e.g. telephone hot-line)		+	+		+[c]
11. Involvement of other family member (e.g. mother-in-law)				+	
12. Positive impact on breast feeding duration	+	+	+[b]		+
13. Reduction in infant morbidity and mortality			+		+

Source: Jelliffe and Jelliffe (1988).
[a]Wet-nursing.
[b]Initiation only.
[c]Home visits.

being placed on introducing appropriate information into both medical and primary and secondary school curricula. The aim of the former is to ensure that doctors and nurses are correctly informed of the benefits and techniques of breast feeding and the practices needed to ensure that breast feeding mothers are adequately supported. In Canada, surveyed GPs were particularly keen for information on the possible transfer of drugs into breast milk, nutrition and lactation, and how to combine working with breast feeding (Jelliffe and Jelliffe, 1988).

By introducing modules on infant feeding in school curricula, it is hoped to change attitudes from an early age. Ultimately this might

Table 3.8 Key features of four national programmes to promote breast feeding (mid-1970s to mid-1980s)

Feature	Brazil	Honduras	Indonesia	Philippines
Interagency task force established	+	+	+	+
Educational/promotional activities targeted at				
– health sector	+	+	+	+
– mothers	+		+	
– schoolchildren	+	+	(+)	(+)
– community (mass media)	+	+	+	+
Changes in health sector practices introduced	+	+	+	+
Support groups set up (e.g. La Leche League/mothers' groups)	+	(+)	+	+
Adoption of WHO/national code on the promotion of breast milk substitutes	+	(a)	(b)	+
Evaluation				
– impact on breast feeding practices	+	+	+[c]	+[c]

Source: Jelliffe and Jelliffe (1988).
(+) Planned activity, (a) approved, awaiting legislation, (b) some of the Code enacted.
[c]Implicit, not formally evaluated but an increase in breast feeding initiation/duration observed.

be expected to lead to a shift away from culturally shaped negative perceptions of breast feeding, for example that it is distasteful or embarrassing (some Western societies) or primitive and old-fashioned (some Third World societies), as well as to dispel commonly held misconceptions about the lactation process. The role of the mass media has not been carefully evaluated.

National support groups, such as La Leche League, with local representation, may exert an important influence on breast feeding rates. In Australia, where a major resurgence of breast feeding has been seen, the Nursing Mothers' Association of Australia is very active: for example, in 1985 the Association received 275 000 telephone requests for information and help, approximately equal to the number of new births per year (Jelliffe and Jelliffe, 1988).

Other programmes may also impact on breast feeding practices: for example, it has been suggested that the recently observed increase in breast feeding duration in Jakarta, Indonesia, may have been influenced by a vigorous national family planning programme. As breast feeding during pregnancy is culturally unacceptable, the increased use of contraceptives may have facilitated prolonged breast feeding. It is interesting to note that the increase in breast feeding has occurred among poorer women where such taboos might be expected to be strongest (Joesoef *et al.* 1989).

Increasingly, national breast feeding promotion programmes are being systematically evaluated. In Brazil and Honduras, for example, baseline and post-intervention data have provided convincing evidence that the programmes have made a significant impact. In Honduras, the PRO-ALMA programme was initiated in 1982, focusing on changing health professionals' knowledge and attitudes about breast feeding. An evaluation of the first 5 years of the programme has been completed using data from three comparable national surveys, a KAP (knowledge–attitudes–practice) survey of health professionals, and community surveys in 19 low-income neighbourhoods served by a teaching hospital. Both initiation and duration of breast feeding increased between 1981 and 1987, with the greatest increase occurring in urban areas in the first half of the study period. In addition, a greater proportion of doctors and nurses responded appropriately to questions relating to practices supportive of breast feeding in 1985 compared with 1982 (Popkin *et al.* 1991).

In Brazil, 6 years after a broad-based national breast feeding programme was launched in 1981, an initial evaluation in São Paulo has shown that the average duration of breast feeding increased from 89 to 127 days. Exclusive breast feeding increased in mean duration from 43 to 67 days and the proportion of children breast fed for more then 6 months increased from 19% for those born in 1981–1982 to 38% for those born in 1984 when programme activities were at their height. By 1985–1986, however, only 28% of children were being breast fed to 6 months. The programme had no significant impact on the initiation of breast feeding, which was already fairly high and rose from 91% to 95% over the study period (Rea and Berquó, 1990).

The Brazilian programme began first with a mass media campaign, followed by further messages delivered by celebrities together with stricter controls on the advertising of breast milk substitutes. In the third phase, training of health professionals took place, but this was followed by a reduction in coordinated activities nationally, which may have contributed to the failure to sustain the initial improvements in duration. A unique feature of the Brazilian programme was its attempt to enforce existing employment legislation guaranteeing working mothers' rights.

It is worth looking in more detail at the Western Australian experience where the role model of the 'élite mother as trend-setter' appears to have held true. Not only were there active support groups and a committed health policy for hospitals and child health centres, dating back to the early 1970s, of encouraging breast feeding for at least 6 months, but also local media gave considerable coverage to related research that was being carried out in Western Australia at that time. A study of information sources showed that the clinic nurse, followed by written materials (books, magazines and pamphlets), were the most important sources for mothers from higher social groups, while the clinic nurse, then family and friends, were most important for lower social groups (Hitchcock and Coy, 1988).

In summary, in designing appropriate messages for breast feeding promotion, it is important to consider the sociocultural background of the groups who are abandoning breast feeding. In the West these are the less educated, poorer women who may be less confident of their own family role and who are eager to accelerate the growth of their children, whereas those choosing to breast feed tend to be better educated, middle to upper class, feel secure about their sexuality and their relationship with their infant's father, and opt for a less interventionist role in terms of infant growth (Kocturk and Zetterstrom, 1989). In the Third World it is the more affluent, better educated women who are abandoning breast feeding. For these, formula feeding may be convenient and perceived as progressive.

It is apparent that, in the context of both developing and Western countries, the health sector plays a pivotal role in influencing infant feeding practices, and that even where no other intervention takes place changes in health worker attitudes and health sector routines can have a major impact on breast feeding. Where this is reinforced by positive messages from other influential sources, the outcome, as in Brazil and Western Australia, can be quite dramatic.

CONCLUSIONS

In this chapter we have focused on breast feeding because of its major contribution to infant health and well-being. We have looked at current patterns of infant feeding and their determinants, and at recent measures adopted either locally or nationally to promote and support breast feeding. From these, a range of interventions may be proposed which, if targeted appropriately, might be expected to have an impact on breast feeding (Table 3.9). While common themes run across the various cultural and social divides, such as concerns over insufficient milk, ignorance as to how to cope with breast problems and so on, it is essential that the local context, including the major constraints faced by mothers, is properly assessed, so that messages are given in the right order of priority and in a culturally appropriate form. Some of the key messages that have emerged from the studies and programmes discussed above are shown in Fig. 3.1. It is important that messages directed to mothers are conveyed in a supportive way and that those who choose, for whatever reason, not to breast feed are not made to feel guilty or inadequate.

Table 3.9 Targeting of interventions to promote breast feeding

Target group	Intervention	Objective
1. Health sector	Education of staff at all levels on the benefits of breast feeding and how to support breast feeding in their institution/community	To achieve changes in knowledge, attitudes and practice; to provide an environment in health facilities conducive to breast feeding; to be role models
2. Preadolescent/adolescent boys and girls; (general public)	Education on the *benefits* of breast feeding and the disbenefits of feeding with infant formula	To change attitudes; to provide sound knowledge and to bring about a change in the cultural perception of breast feeding
3. (a) Pregnant women and their partners/ other influential individuals (NB: single low-income mothers particularly at risk in Western countries)	Education on the *benefits* of breast feeding and the disbenefits of feeding with infant formula. Education on the *techniques* of breast feeding: how to overcome problems likely to be encountered, e.g. crying, sore nipples	To encourage breast feeding and allay anxiety and facili- tate a relaxed, enjoyable breast feeding experience
(b) Breast feeding mothers	Advice/counselling as above, also on how to cope with breast feeding and employment	To provide continuing support to the breast feeding mother and enable her to breast feed for as long as possible
4. Government/employers opinion-formers, e.g mass media	Education on the benefits of breast feeding (including socioeconomic) Lobbying on: (1) Changes in maternity/ paternity leave allowances; other employment legislation related to facilities at work, etc.	To provide sound arguments for a change in legis- lation so that working mothers are able to breast feed for as long as possible
	(2) Enforcement of the WHO code restricting the promotion of breast milk substitutes	To ensure that counter-messages on breast feeding substitutes are not disseminated through any agency or mass media

MESSAGES   TARGETS

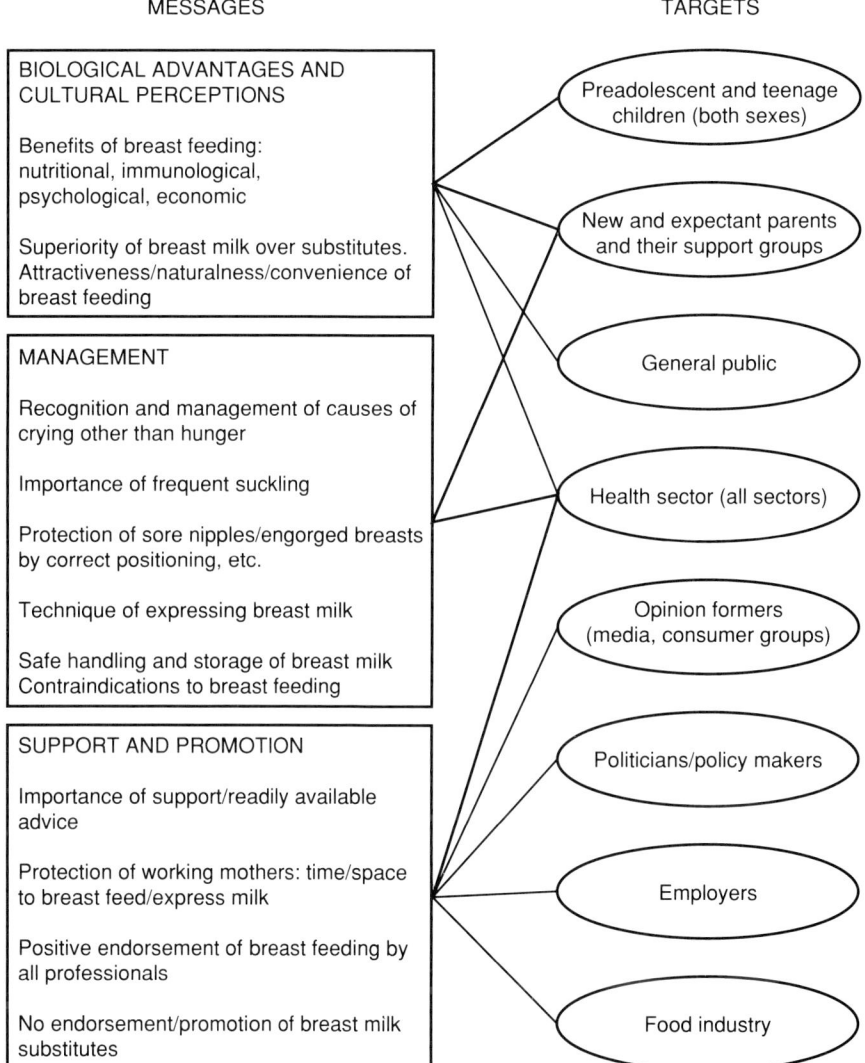

Figure 3.1 Important breast feeding messages and their main targets.

Timely and nutritious weaning foods to supplement and eventually substitute for breast milk are of paramount importance. In the Third World
context, there is an urgent need to promote the use of weaning foods with
a high nutritional value, which can be prepared safely and which are made
from cheap local ingredients. This issue is discussed in greater detail in
Chapter 9. Here again, the health sector and mass media can play a major

role. There has been little focus so far on weaning practices in Western countries and, given the possible long-term effects of early diet on health and development (Barker *et al.* 1989), this is an area that warrants further study.

Further studies are needed into the best means of ensuring effective communication between health professionals and the community they serve. The development of such a dialogue as an ongoing process, responding to changing socioeconomic and cultural needs and constraints, would ensure a flexible and appropriate approach to promoting and supporting the best possible infant feeding practices under the prevailing circumstances.

Tables 3.7 and 3.8 present evidence that both local and national pro-motional campaigns can be effective. National programmes have an important role in ensuring that the necessary changes to traditional health service routines take place and that consistent messages are conveyed to all target groups. Such programmes require governmental commitment, not only to promoting breast feeding but also to withstanding the pres-sures from the powerful infant food industry lobby. Operational targets in the Innocenti Declaration (1990) specify that all governments by the year 1995 should have:

1. appointed a national breast feeding coordinator and established a multisectoral national breast feeding committee representing relevant government departments, non-governmental organizations and health professional associations;
2. ensured that every maternity facility fully practises the Ten Steps to Successful Breast-feeding (WHO, 1989b);
3. taken action to give effect to the principles and aims of all the Articles of the WHO Code in their entirety;
4. enacted imaginative legislation protecting the breast feeding rights of working women and established means for its enforcement.

All governments are further urged to develop national breast feeding policies and set national targets for the 1990s, establish a national moni-toring system, and develop indicators such as the prevalence of exclusively breast-fed infants at discharge from the maternity centre, and the preva-lence at 4 months post partum. The UK government recently proposed the following targets for breast feeding in England: 'to increase the pro-portion nationally of infants who are breast-fed at birth from 64% in 1985 to 75% by 2000; and to increase the proportion of infants nationally aged 6 weeks being wholly or partly breast-fed from 39% to 50% by 2000' (HMSO, 1991).

These are worthwhile targets and there is now a need to define the most appropriate and effective measures to be adopted to ensure that they are met.

REFERENCES

Auerbach, K.G. and Guss, E. (1984) Maternal employment and breast-feeding. *American Journal of Diseases in Childhood* **138**, 958–960.

Barker, D.J.P., Osmond, C. and Law, C.M. (1989) The intrauterine and early postnatal origins of cardiovascular disease and chronic bronchitis. *Journal of Epidemiology and Community Health*, **43**, 237–240.

Bauchner, H., Leventhal, J.M. and Shapiro, E.D. (1986) Studies of breast-feeding and infections: how good is the evidence? *Journal of the American Medical Association*, **256**, 887–892.

Bryant, C.A. (1982) The impact of kin, friend and neighbour networks on infant feeding practices. *Social Science and Medicine*, **16**, 1757–1765.

Butz, W.P. (1977) Economic aspects of breastfeeding. *The Rand Paper Series*, P-*5801*. Santa Monica: Rand Corporation.

Carballo, M. and Pelto, G. (1991) Social and psychological factors in breast-feeding. In *Infant Feeding and Child Nutrition: Issues and Perspectives*, pp. 177–192 (ed. F. Falkner). Boca Raton, FL: CRC Press.

Cardenas, A.M., Gonzalas, L.M.P., Garcia de Alba, J.E. *et al.* (1981) Some epidemiological aspects of maternal breast-feeding in a population entitled to social welfare services in Mexico. *Bulletin of the Pan American Health Organization*, **15**, 139–147.

Cunningham, W.E. and Segree, W. (1990) Breast-feeding promotion in an urban and a rural Jamaican hospital. *Social Science and Medicine*, **30**, 341–348.

Dimond, H.J. and Ashworth, A. (1987) Infant feeding practices in Kenya, Mexico and Malaysia: the rarity of the exclusively breast-fed infant. *Human Nutrition, Applied Nutrition*, **41A**, 51–64.

Feinstein, J.M., Berkelhauer, J.G., Gruszka, M.E. *et al.* (1986) Factors related to early termination of breast-feeding in an urban population. *Pediatrics*, **78**, 210–215.

Ferry, B. (1981) Breast-feeding. *World Fertility Survey Comparative Studies no. 13.* The Hague: International Statistics Institute.

Frank, D.A., Wirtz, S.J., Sorenson, J.R. and Heeren, T. (1987) Commercial discharge packs and breast-feeding counselling: effects on infant feeding practices in a randomized trial. *Pediatrics*, **80**, 845–853.

Gabriel, A., Gabriel, K.R. and Lawrence, R.A. (1986) Cultural values and biomedical knowledge: choices in infant feeding. *Social Science and Medicine*, **23**, 501–509.

Gussler, J.D. and Mock, N. (1983) A comparative description of infant feeding practices in Zaire, the Philippines and St Kitts–Nevis. *Ecology of Food and Nutrition*, **13**, 75–85.

Haaga, J.G. (1986) Evidence of a reversal of the breast-feeding decline in peninsular Malaysia. *American Journal of Public Health*, **76**, 245–251.

Hanson, L.A. (ed) (1988) *Biology of Human Milk.* Nestlé Nutrition Workshop Series no. 15. New York: Raven Press.

Hitchcock, N.E. and Coy, J.F. (1988) Infant feeding practices in Western Australia and Tasmania: a joint survey 1984–85. *Medical Journal of Public Health*, **148**, 114–117.

HMSO (1991) *The Health of the Nation. A Consultative Document for Health in England.* Presented to Parliament by the Secretary of State of Health. Cmnd 1523. London: HMSO.

Hull, V.G., Thapa, S. and Wiknjosastro, G. (1989) Breast-feeding and health professionals: a study in hospitals in Indonesia. *Social Science and Medicine*, **28**, 355–364.

Innocenti Declaration (1990) Adopted at the WHO/UNICEF policymakers' meeting on *Breast-feeding in the 1990s: A Global Initiative*, held in Florence, Italy, 30 July–1 August 1990. New York: UNICEF.

Jelliffe, D. and Jelliffe, E. (eds) (1988) *Programmes to Promote Breast-feeding.* New York: Oxford University Press.

Joesoef, M.R., Annest, J.L. and Utomo, B. (1989) A recent increase of breast-feeding duration in Jakarta, Indonesia. *American Journal of Public Health*, **79**, 36–38.

King, J. and Ashworth, A. (1987) Historical review of the changing pattern of infant feeding in developing countries: the case of Malaysia, the Caribbean, Nigeria and Zaire. *Social Science and Medicine*, **25**, 1307–1320.

King, J. and Ashworth, A. (1991) Contemporary feeding practices in infancy and early childhood in developing countries. In *Infant Feeding and Child Nutrition: Issues and Perspectives*, pp. 143–176 (ed F. Falkner). Boca Raton, FL: CRC Press.

Kocturk, T. and Zetterstrom, R. (1989) The promotion of breast-feeding and maternal attitudes. *Acta Paediatrica Scandinavica*, **78**, 817–823.

Kurinij, N., Shiona, P.H., Ezrine, S.F. and Rhoads, G.G. (1989) Does maternal employment affect breast-feeding? *American Journal of Public Health*, **79**, 1247–1250.

Lawrence, R.A. and Friedman, L.R. (1990) Breast-feeding practices in industrialized countries. In *Breast-feeding, Nutrition, Infection and Infant Growth in Developed and Emerging Countries*, pp. 447–455 (eds S.A. Atkinson, L.A. Hanson and R.K. Chandra). St John's, Newfoundland: ARTS Biomedical Publishers.

Leslie, J. (1985) *Women's Work and Child Nutrition in the Third World.* Paper presented at a Policy Conference, International Center for Research on Women, Washington, DC, November 3.

Martin, J. (1978) *Infant Feeding 1975: Attitudes and Practices in England and Wales.* Office of Population Censuses and Surveys. London: HMSO.

Martin, J. and Monk, J. (1982) *Infant Feeding 1980.* Office of Population Censuses and Surveys. London: HMSO.

Martin, J. and White, A. (1988) *Infant Feeding 1985.* Office of Population Censuses and Surveys. London: HMSO.

Martinez, G.A. and Krieger, F.W. (1985) 1984 Milk-feeding patterns in the United States. *Pediatrics*, **76**, 1004–1008.

Oppé, T.E. (1974) *Present Day Practices in Infant Feeding.* Report of a Working Party of the Panel on Child Nutrition, Committee on Medical Aspects of Food Policy (COMA). Department of Health and Social Security Report on Health and Social Subjects no. 9. London: HMSO.

Palmer, G. (1988) *The Politics of Breast-feeding.* London: Pandora Press.

Popkin, B.M., Bilsborrow, R.E. and Akin, J.S. (1982) Breast-feeding patterns in low-income countries. *Science*, **218**, 1088–1093.

Popkin, B.M., Canahuti, J., Bailey, P.G. and O'Gara, C. (1991) An evaluation of a national breast-feeding promotion programme in Honduras. *Journal of Biosocial Science*, **23**, 5–21.

Rassin, D.K., Richardson, C.J., Baranowski, T. *et al.* (1984) Incidence of breast-feeding in a low socio-economic group of mothers in the United States: ethnic patterns. *Pediatrics*, **73**, 132–137.

Rea, M.F. and Berquó, E.S. (1990) Impact of the Brazilian national breast-feeding programme on mothers in Greater São Paulo. *Bulletin of the World Health Organization*, **68**, 365–371.

Reiff, M.I. and Essock-Vitale, S.M. (1985) Hospital influences on early infant feeding practices. *Pediatrics*, **76**, 872–879.

Ryan, A.S. and Martinez, G.A. (1989) Breast-feeding and the working mother: a profile. *Pediatrics*, **83**, 524–531.

Winikoff, B. and Laukaran, V.H. (1989) Breast-feeding and bottle-feeding controversies in the developing world: evidence from a study in four countries. *Social Science and Medicine*, **29**, 859–868.

Winikoff, B., Laukaran, V.H., Myers, D. and Stone, R. (1986) Dynamics of infant feeding: mothers, professionals and the institutional context in a large urban hospital. *Pediatrics*, **77**, 357–365.

Winikoff, B., Myers, D., Laukaran, V.H. and Stone, R. (1987) Overcoming obstacles to breast-feeding in a large municipal hospital: applications of lessons learned. *Pediatrics*, **80**, 423–433.

WHO (1981) Contemporary Patterns of Breast-feeding. *Report of the WHO Collaborative Study on Breast-feeding.* Geneva: World Health Organization.

WHO (1982) The prevalence and duration of breast-feeding: a critical review of available information. *WHO Statistics Quarterly*, **35**, 92–116.

WHO (1989a) The prevalence and duration of breast-feeding: updated information, 1980–89; Part II. *Weekly Epidemiological Record*, **64**, 331–335.

WHO (1989b) *Protecting, Promoting and Supporting Breast-feeding: The Special Role of Maternity Services.* Geneva: World Health Organization.

4
Perinatal development of digestive enzymes

Jacques Riby

Department of Nutritional Sciences, University of California, USA

INTRODUCTION

All mammals have a pattern of perinatal physiological development that is partly influenced by exposure to the extrauterine environment. At birth, the newborn can no longer rely on placental exchange for its nutrition, thus making it dependent on absorption and digestion of nutrients via its own gastrointestinal tract. Maternal milk is generally the only source of nutrients during the suckling period (Fig. 4.1) and the digestive capabilities of the gastrointestinal tract are correspondingly specialized (Doell and Kretchmer, 1962; Sunshine *et al.* 1971). As the animal is weaned from milk and other foods are introduced (Fig. 4.2), the gastro-intestinal tract again undergoes profound changes (Henning, 1981; Kretchmer, 1985). The ontogeny of the mammalian gastrointestinal tract from the embryo to the adult has been studied extensively and is the subject of several exhaustive publications describing the structural and the metabolic aspects of the maturation (Henning and Kretchmer, 1973; Grand *et al.* 1976; Lebenthal, 1981, 1989; Klein and McKenzie, 1983; Henning, 1985, 1987).

This chapter will review the development of the enzymes of the gastro-intestinal tract responsible for the digestion and absorption of the three basic groups of nutrients: protein, carbohydrate and fat. Morphological changes occurring during development and the changes in other function-al aspects such as gut motility or gastric emptying are beyond the scope of

Infant Nutrition. Edited by A.F. Walker and B.A. Rolls.
Published in 1994 by Chapman & Hall, London.
ISBN 0 412 59140 5.

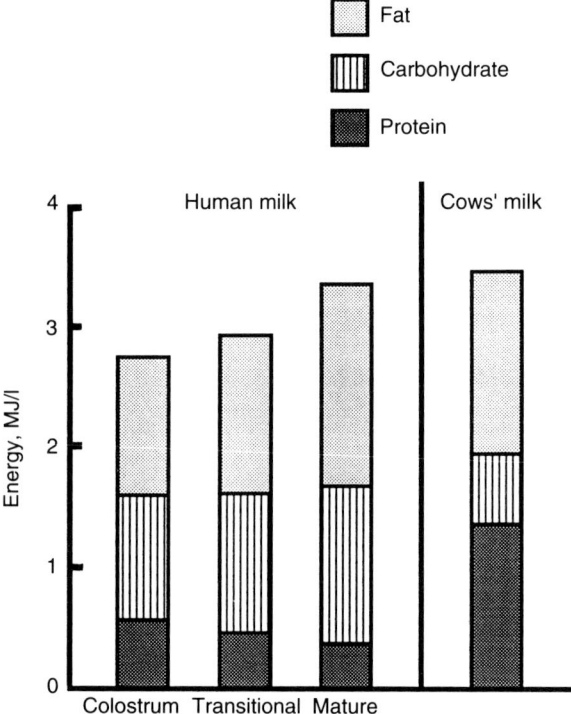

Figure 4.1 Composition of human milk and cows' milk: colostrum, first 5 days post partum; transitional milk, 6–14 days post partum; mature milk, 15 days post partum to end of lactation. (Data from Dieu and Lentner, 1970.)

the present chapter and will be mentioned only when necessary for comprehension. Regulatory control of the development of digestive functions has been studied almost exclusively in animal models (Doell and Kretchmer, 1962; Sunshine *et al.* 1971; Henning and Kretchmer, 1973; Henning, 1981, 1985; Klein and McKenzie, 1983; Kretchmer, 1985) and information derived from clinical observations is very limited. Because of the fundamental differences in the timing of physiological events in different species, maturational changes that take place in the human will be discussed comparatively to that encountered in other animals.

Lactose intolerance is a particular situation deserving additional attention and will be discussed in a separate section at the end of the chapter.

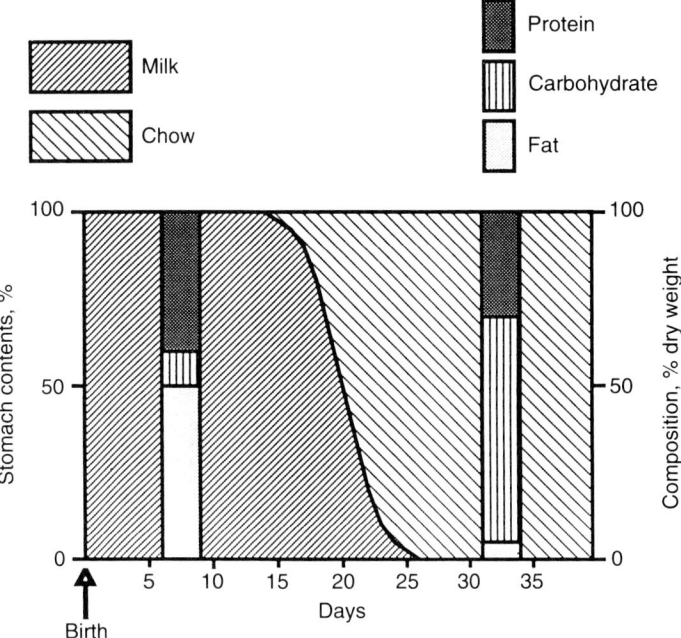

Figure 4.2 Changes in the composition of the diet of the rat at weaning. (Data from Dymsza *et al.* 1964, and Henning *et al.* 1979.)

PROTEIN DIGESTION

The digestion of proteins involves two complementary physiological components: intraluminal digestion and mucosal digestion. Intraluminal digestion consists of gastric proteolysis by the enzyme pepsin in the acidic environment of the stomach followed by intestinal proteolysis by the pancreatic enzymes excreted into the lumen of the duodenum. Pancreatic proteolytic enzymes are excreted in the form of inactive precursors: trypsinogen, chymotrypsinogen, procarboxypeptidases A and B and proelastase (Figs 4.3 and 4.4). The duodenal brush border enteropeptidase (enterokinase) activates trypsin by proteolytic cleavage of a short peptide of six amino acids from the precursor trypsinogen. Trypsin activates the other proteinases by similar proteolytic cleavage.

The short peptides and free amino acids resulting from luminal digestion of dietary protein are then further digested and absorbed by the intestinal mucosa (Fig. 4.5). Small peptides consisting of two or three amino acids are mostly (80–90%) absorbed intact by the epithelial cell and hydrolysed by intracellular dipeptidases and tripeptidases. The remaining oligopeptides and larger peptides are hydrolysed by enzymes

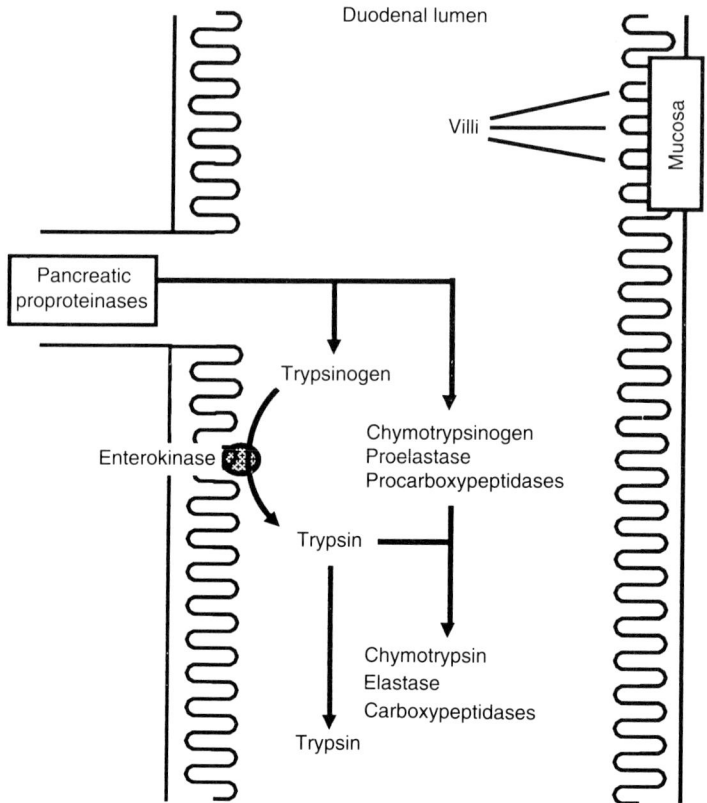

Figure 4.3 Activation of pancreatic proteinases.

that are integral parts of the microvillous (brush border) membrane, and the resultant amino acids are absorbed directly through the membrane.

Development of intraluminal proteolysis

In the human fetus, hydrochloric acid and pepsin have been found in the stomach at 12 and 34 weeks of gestation respectively, but the concentrations measured in the term infant are still insufficient to account for any substantial amount of proteolysis (Hadorn, 1981). Analyses of the gastric contents of the newborn sampled 3 hours after a meal of maternal milk have shown that the protein micelles were still intact. Pepsin and HCl concentration in the stomach increase proportionately with the gain in body weight during the first 4 months after birth (Deren, 1971). It has been suggested, however, that even in adults peptic proteolysis may not

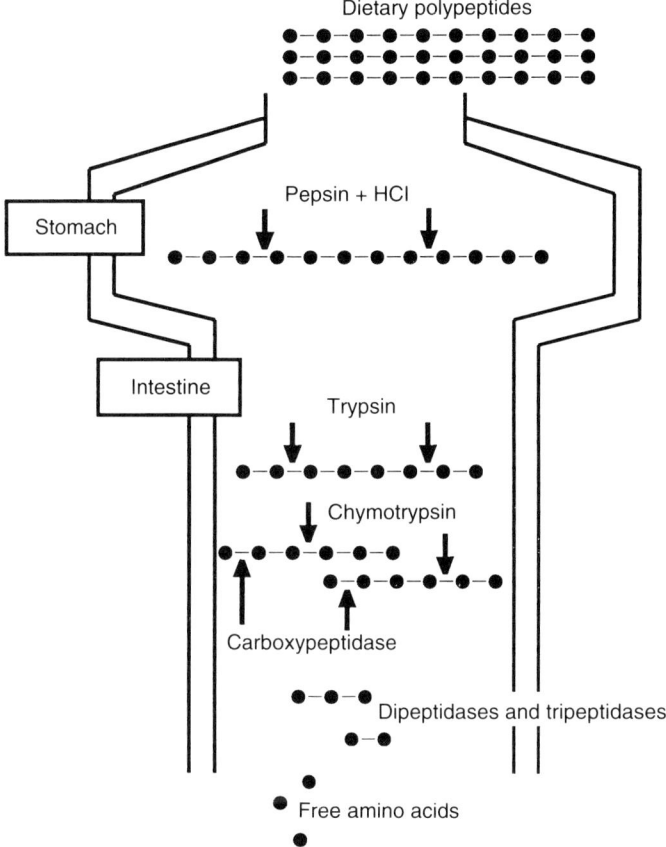

Figure 4.4 Luminal digestion of proteins.

contribute significantly to protein digestion since gastrectomy does not effectively impair protein absorption (Taylor, 1968).

The precursors of pancreatic proteolytic enzymes are found in zymogen granules at as early as 12 weeks of gestation and at 26 weeks enterokinase is present in the duodenal mucosa (Hadorn, 1981). At birth exocrine pancreatic secretion of proteolytic enzymes is fully developed (Henning, 1987). There is evidence that during the last several weeks of gestation the pancreatic proteolysis actually processes proteins that are ingested by the fetus with the amniotic fluid: in newborns with early signs of cystic fibrosis (resulting in insufficient exocrine pancreatic function) or in pre-term infants, the meconium (intestinal contents of the newborn) contains higher concentrations of albumin than in healthy full-term infants (Hadorn, 1981).

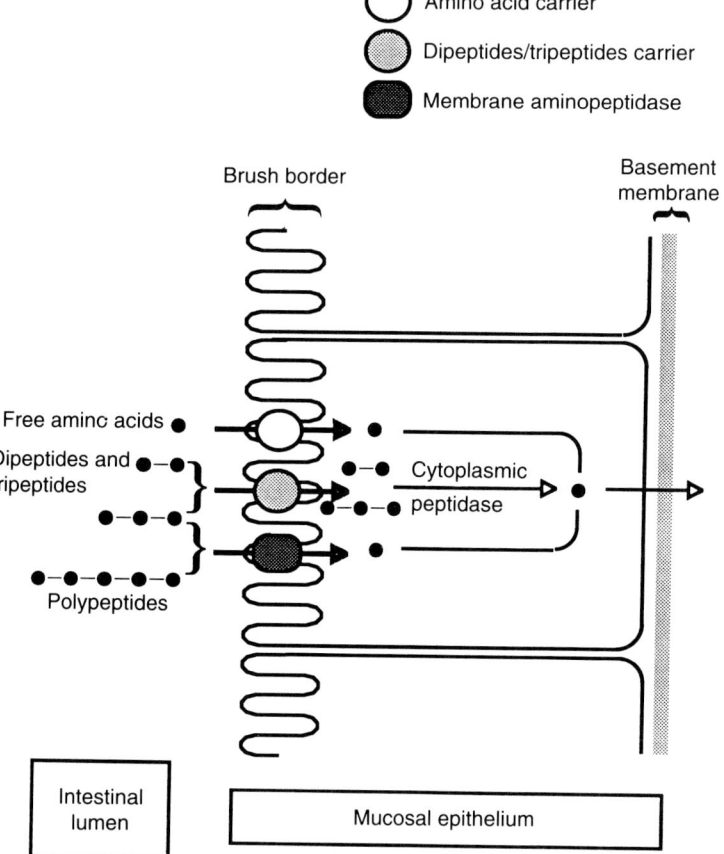

Figure 4.5 Mucosal digestion and absorption of peptides.

Development of mucosal absorption of amino acids and peptides

The development of small intestinal transport of free amino acids and of dipeptides and tripeptides has been studied only in animals: in rabbits transport of free amino acids is detected early in the fetal intestine and it is elevated in the neonate compared with the adult. Development of the transport of intact dipeptides and tripeptides follows the same pattern: it first appears at 25 days of gestation, reaches a peak at birth, declines progressively through the suckling period and is comparable to that of the adult after weaning is completed (Auricchio *et al.* 1981). The development of cytosolic small intestinal dipeptidases has been studied in the human fetus but not during the perinatal period: activity is already present at 11 weeks of gestation and reaches adult values by 14 weeks (Auricchio *et al.* 1981). In rats there is a peak of activity at birth followed by a decline to adult values at weaning. In addition, in these animal studies, both the transport of intact peptides and the subsequent cytosolic peptidase activity followed the same developmental pattern, indicating that this function is well developed at birth.

Peptidases bound to the brush border membrane also appear early during gestation in humans and reach adult levels at various times before birth. Aminopeptidase A is an exception since it reaches only a quarter of adult activity at birth. Postnatal development of membrane-bound peptidases has been studied only in rats. The activity of individual enzymes increases at different rates, but the general pattern is a peak of activity during the suckling period with a decline to adult activity by the end of weaning (Auricchio *et al.* 1981).

The gastrointestinal tract of the human neonate possesses all the necessary enzymes, and dietary protein and peptides can be digested as effectively as in the adult (Hadorn, 1981; Henning, 1981, 1987; Kretchmer, 1985). In contrast, in the rat peptic secretion and pancreatic exocrine proteolysis do not develop until weaning, and alimentary proteins reach the ileum intact with no luminal degradation. During the suckling period pinocytotic activity is still very active in the small intestine of the rat (Henning, 1981, 1987; Lebenthal, 1981). Immunoglobulins, a significant part of milk proteins, are transported intact through the mucosa of the jejunum to the circulatory system of the newborn rat. In the mucosa of the ileum, proteins absorbed by pinocytosis are degraded by lysosomal proteinases (cathepsin B). Closure of the small intestinal epithelium of the rat to the transport of intact proteins happens at weaning simultaneously with the decline of lysosomal proteolytic activity and with the maturation of the enzymes required for luminal proteolysis. In the human newborn, milk immunoglobulins (mostly of the IgA class) are not transported to the circulatory system in any large amounts but play their defensive function in the lumen of the intestine (Walker, 1985). Human milk immunoglobulins are very resistant to proteolysis and account for the high nitrogen content in the faeces of the newborn. Some dietary proteins, immunoglobulins and others, have been detected in the plasma of infants, especially in cases where the gastrointestinal mucosa was immature or damaged, such as in pre-term or malnourished infants but also in healthy full-term infants. This can be perceived as a continuation of the fetal absorptive process in which absorption of macromolecules is very active. However, it does not constitute a significant mode of absorption of dietary protein by the human newborn in contrast to what was found in the rat (Walker, 1985).

CARBOHYDRATE DIGESTION

Milk is the only source of lactose. In human milk, lactose accounts for approximately one-third of the total energy (Fig. 4.1). Only trace amounts of monosaccharides such as glucose and fructose and nucleotide sugars such as fucose are present in milk (Walker, 1985). Small quantities of glycolipids and glycoproteins are also found, but these are not considered a part of the dietary carbohydrate. In addition to maternal milk, human infants may receive artificial formulas or solid foods (liquefied meat or vegetable products) soon after birth. The carbohydrate content of these products is as complex as that of post-weaning diets, and it is therefore necessary to know the developmental patterns of the various digestive processes involved in order to understand the ability of the newborn to thrive under these conditions.

Absorption of monosaccharides

An active transport system has been shown to be responsible for absorption of glucose and galactose in the small intestine (Fig. 4.6). The carrier is a protein of the brush border membrane that can transfer one molecule of glucose or (galactose) and one atom of sodium simultaneously, from the luminal side of the membrane to the cytoplasmic side. The system is driven by the negative gradient of the concentration of sodium between the lumen and the cell. The low intracellular concentration of sodium is maintained by the Na$^+$ATPase of the basolateral membrane, and this constitutes the energy-dependent part of the process. Binding of glucose to the active site of the carrier is inhibited by the glucoside phlorizin (Crane, 1975). Active transport of glucose and galactose was demonstrated *in vitro* in isolated segments of fetal intestine beginning at 10 weeks of gestation and increasing to the adult level at 18 weeks (Younoszai, 1974). Measurements of the rate of absorption using perfusion of the intestine *in vivo* show significant absorption of glucose although at slower rates in infants than in adults. Rates of absorption equal to those in adults were reached in children at approximately 5 years of age (Younoszai, 1974).

Fructose absorption is not dependent on sodium and is not inhibited by phlorizin. Facilitated diffusion is the mechanism generally accepted, because fructose is absorbed at a slower rate than glucose or galactose but faster than mannitol, a compound known to be absorbed by passive diffusion. Kinetics show that absorption is mediated by a carrier (Sigrist-Nelson and Hopfer, 1974). Absorption of fructose was shown to be dependent on a supply of oxygen *in vitro*, suggesting that a component of the mechanism of transport might be of the active type (Gracey *et al.* 1970).

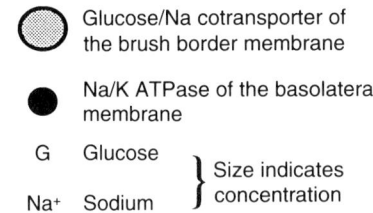

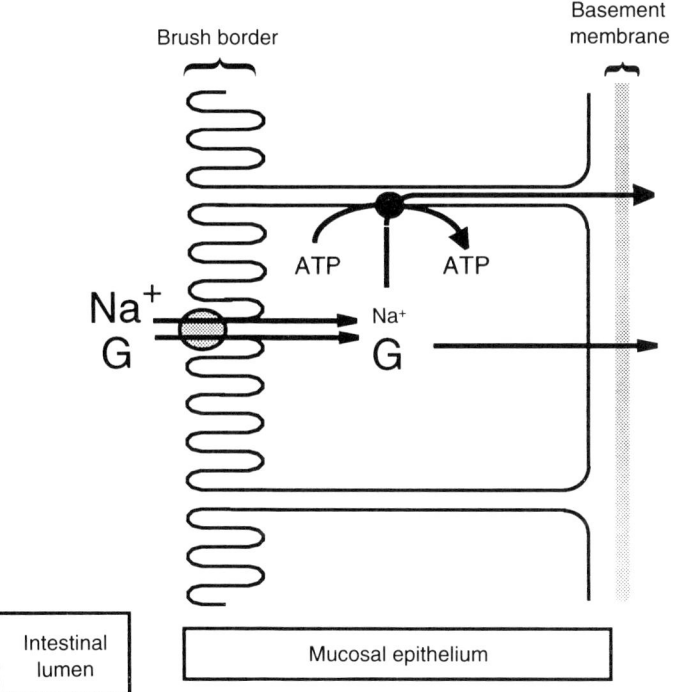

Figure 4.6 Active transport of glucose in the epithelial cells of the intestine.

Digestion of disaccharides

Most of the dietary carbohydrates reach the intestinal mucosa in the form of disaccharides. Lactose and sucrose, the main disaccharides in the diet, are not affected by salivary, gastric or pancreatic enzymes and reach the small intestine intact. Maltose is the product of the luminal digestion of large dietary polysaccharides, starch and glycogen, by salivary and pancreatic α-amylase (Figs 4.7 and 4.8). Digestion of the branched polysaccharides amylopectin and glycogen also produces isomaltose.

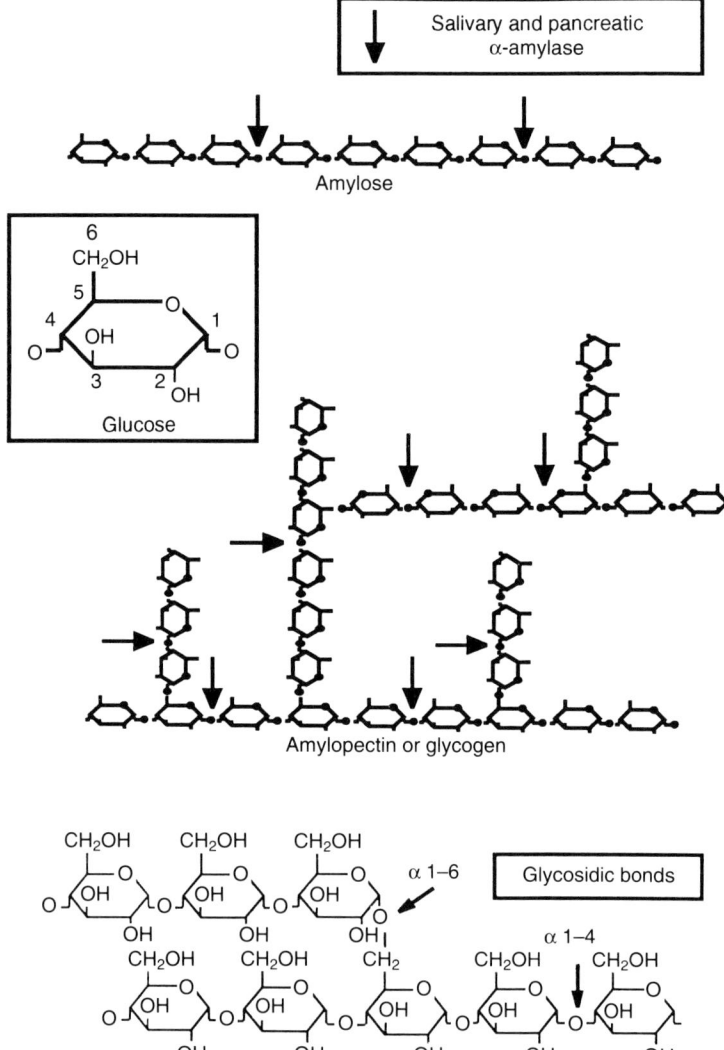

Figure 4.7 Luminal digestion of polysaccharides.

Other carbohydrates present in the intestinal lumen include trehalose, a disaccharide found primarily in mushrooms and insects, and various oligosaccharides and indigestible fibres such as cellulose.

The small intestinal mucosa of most mammals possesses the following disaccharidase activities: lactase, sucrase, maltase, isomaltase and trehalase. Four enzyme complexes responsible for these activities were found in

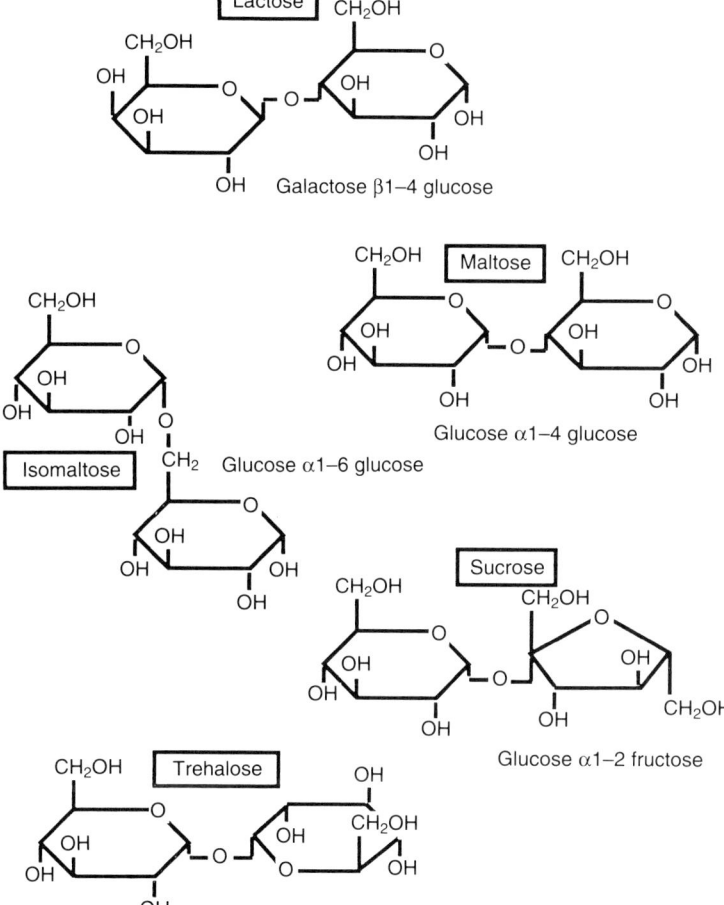

Figure 4.8 Disaccharides.

the membrane of the brush border of the enterocyte (Semenza, 1986).

Lactase–phlorizin hydrolase is a dimeric enzyme, comprising two sub-units. The active sites of both subunits have a broad specificity and will use as a substrate a variety of β-glycosides, of which lactose is the only one with significant nutritional importance. It has been suggested that phlorizin hydrolase activity could play a role in the dispersion of milk fat globules by hydrolysing the glycosyl-ceramides that are components of the membrane of the globules.

Sucrase–isomaltase is also a dimeric enzyme and the two subunits have active sites with different substrate specificity. One hydrolyses maltose and sucrose and the other hydrolyses maltose and isomaltose. Even though these are primarily maltases they were named sucrase and isomaltase in order to distinguish them from the next complex.

Maltase–glucoamylase possesses two subunits with identical substrate specificity. Both active sites hydrolyse maltose and longer glucose polymers with 1–4 glycosidic bonds, releasing one unit at a time from the end of the linear chain.

Trehalase is different from the other disaccharidases in several ways. Its substrate specificity is strictly limited to trehalose, a disaccharide made of two glucose moieties with a glycosidic bond in the 1–1 configuration. It is unclear whether it has one or several subunits. In addition, the hydrophobic nature of trehalase seems to indicate that it is more deeply embedded into the lipid bilayer of the brush border membrane than the other disaccharidases.

With the exception of trehalase, disaccharidases were found to possess large hydrophilic domains that protrude into the intestinal lumen (Fig. 4.9). The disaccharide substrate is captured by the active site on the luminal side of the membrane and the two monosaccharide products of the enzymic hydrolysis are transferred directly across the membrane by a transporter closely associated with the enzyme, or possibly by the enzyme itself, without mixing with the intraluminal pool of monosaccharides (Semenza, 1986).

Development of disaccharidases

Intestinal disaccharidases best exemplify the early development of the digestive tract of the human newborn, in contrast to that of animal models such as the rat (Fig. 4.10). In all mammals lactase activity appears during fetal development, rises rapidly during late gestation and is at a maximum around birth (Doell and Kretchmer, 1962; Grand *et al.* 1976; Mobassaleh *et al.* 1985). In humans, intestinal lactase activity is first detected at 3 months of gestation but does not rise significantly until the last few weeks preceding birth (Grand *et al.* 1976). Pre-term infants are often unable to digest lactose completely and have to receive an alternative source of carbohydrate either enterally or by intravenous feeding until they have developed sufficient lactase activity to be given maternal milk or a lactose-based formula. The change in activity of lactase during childhood and into adulthood varies markedly among individuals and between ethnic groups, as we shall see in the section concerning lactose intolerance: the dominant pattern is a progressive decline in activity. The activity in the adult is only a fraction of the activity found in infants. Some individuals, however, will retain a significant activity even when adult. In other animal species

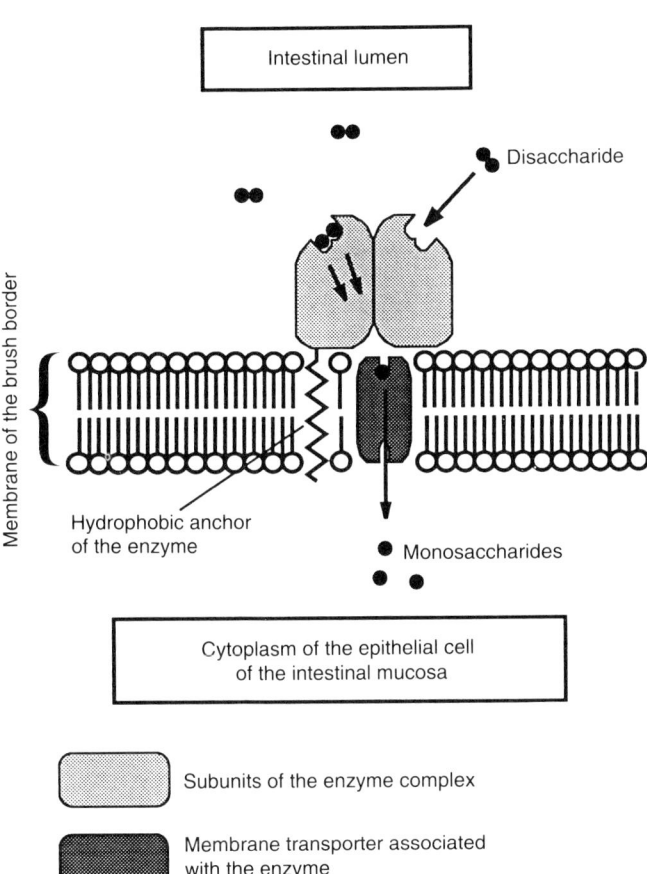

Figure 4.9 Hydrolysis and absorption of disaccharides by the disaccharidases of the brush border.

lactase declines abruptly with weaning when the diet changes from maternal milk to solid food containing other carbohydrates, but no lactose. Although there is no direct association, in rats, mice or rabbits post-weaning lactase activity is approximately one-tenth that of the suckling animal (Mobassaleh *et al.* 1985).

The disaccharidases necessary for digestion of the carbohydrates present in solid food are either absent or extremely low at birth in most mammals (Fig. 4.10). In the rat, maltase activity is very low during the whole suckling period and increases rapidly during weaning, to reach adult activity by the end of the third week of life. Sucrase, isomaltase and trehalase are undetectable at birth, appear suddenly at the beginning of

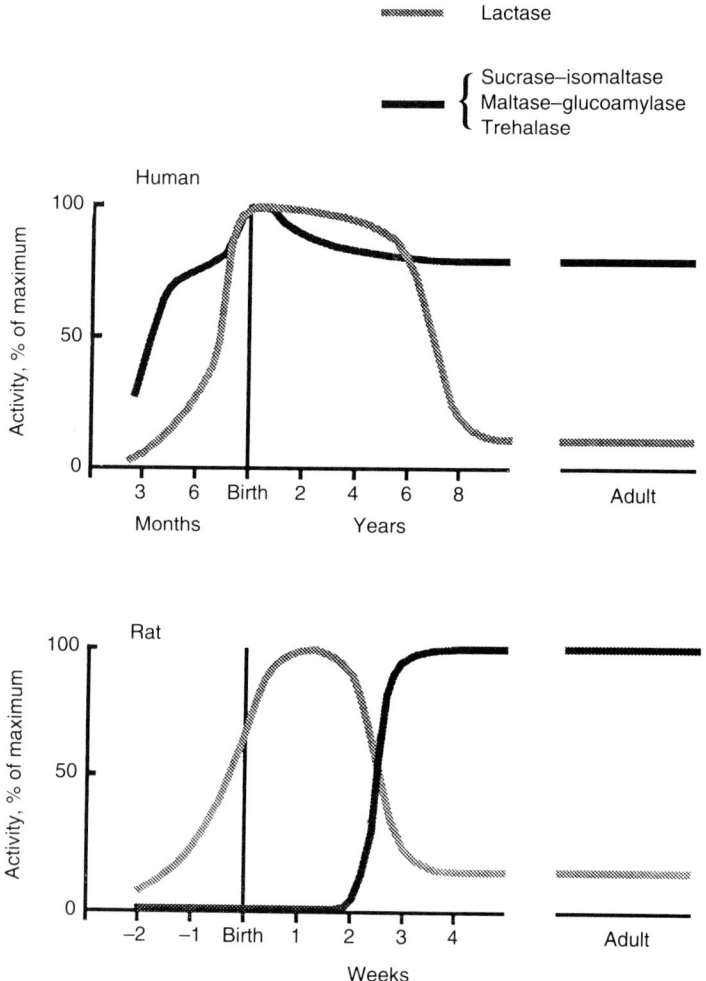

Figure 4.10 Early development of disaccharidases in the human and the rat.

the third week and are at the activity of the adult at the end of weaning. Therefore, in the rat and other animals, there is a high degree of temporal correlation between the development of specific digestive enzymes and the nature of the carbohydrate ingested. In contrast, the development of these disaccharidases in humans shows a different pattern (Grand *et al.* 1976; Mobassaleh *et al.* 1985): sucrase, maltase, trehalase and glucoamylase appear in the fetal intestine during the first trimester of gestation and have activities comparable to those in the adult intestine throughout most of the fetal life. A significant increase during the last trimester leads to a peak of activity at term. The increased activity of glucoamylase in the intestine of full-term infants and also in pre-terms provides an alternative digestive capacity for starches at birth at a time when pancreatic amylase is not yet present. This early development of intestinal disaccharidases makes it possible for the human newborn to thrive on a variety of foods in addition to maternal milk. This may have constituted an evolutionary advantage whenever maternal milk was not available in sufficient quantities or was not well tolerated.

Digestion of starches

Starches are the major source of carbohydrates for children and adults and are remarkably well tolerated. The bioavailability of starch is more of a concern with newborns and infants where undigested carbohydrates could potentially cause diarrhoea. Relative proportions of the two types of glucose polymers, amylose and amylopectin, vary in starches from different plant sources (Fig. 4.7). Amylose is a linear polymer of glucose units linked by α-1,4 glycosidic bonds and amylopectin is a branched polymer with side chains originating with α-1,6 bonds. In natural foods, starches are found as insoluble granules representing a crystalline form of the polymers. Modified food starches are often used in food processing because of their physical properties. Modification is achieved by several chemical manipulations, including replacement of hydroxyl groups by larger substituents and crosslinking between polymers to prevent aggregation and formation of a gel. Baby foods typically contain approximately 5% of modified food starch (Subcommittee on the Evaluation of the Safety of Modified Starches in Infant Foods, 1977). The digestibility of modified starch has not been well established but *in vitro* studies shows that it is resistant to enzymic hydrolysis. The insoluble granular structure of natural starch is destroyed by heating and agitation, making starch in cooked foods accessible to enzymic hydrolysis.

The digestion of starch consists of luminal digestion and mucosal digestion (Mobassaleh *et al.* 1985). Luminal digestion is initiated in the mouth with salivary α-amylase. Acidity and peptic proteolysis partly inactivate salivary amylase during gastric transit but some activity is found in the duodenum. The major source of amylase activity in the intestinal lumen derives from the exocrine pancreas. Pancreatic α-amylase represents 85% of the total amylolytic activity in the duodenum of healthy adults, and 60% in patients with chronic pancreatitis. In the human newborn salivary amylase is fully developed but its actual contribution to digestion of starch is uncertain since it has not been established whether the enzyme reaches the intestinal lumen or is inactivated in the stomach. Pancreatic amylase is undetectable in the duodenal contents of infants during the first 3 months of life even though some amylase activity was found in the fetal pancreas at 22 weeks of gestation, suggesting a lack of secretion (Mobassaleh *et al.* 1985).

Therefore, in the human infant there seems to be little potential for luminal digestion of starch. The exact timing of the development of pancreatic amylase remains to be established, but at 2 years of age the activity is equal to that of the adult. In the rat, neither salivary nor pancreatic α-amylase is present at birth. The activities of both enzymes appear at the end of the second week after birth and reach adult level by the end of weaning, in perfect synchronization with the introduction of starch as the major carbohydrate of the post-weaning diet.

Mucosal digestion of starch is accomplished by the glucoamylase activity of the brush border enzyme, maltase–glucoamylase, described in the section on intestinal disaccharidases. Glucoamylase activity is not essential for the digestion of starch in adults, since most of the starch is reduced to maltose and small glucose oligomers by α-amylases in the lumen before coming into contact with the intestinal mucosa. In human infants, however, glucoamylase may provide an effective route for the digestion of starch in view of the lack of luminal digestion (Raul *et al.* 1986). Foods containing starches, including commercially available baby foods, are commonly given to infants soon after birth with no adverse effects. Studies of starch digestibility in infants have shown a moderate elevation of blood glucose following ingestion of starch (Mobassaleh *et al.* 1985). However, some of the younger subjects (two out of five 1-month-old infants) had diarrhoea when ingesting a small amount of starch (40 g/day), indicating that the intestinal capacity for the digestion of starch is diminished in newborns. A possible explanation is that the amylopectin component of starch cannot be digested by glucoamylase as readily as amylose because of its branched structure. In that respect some starches containing a low proportion of amylopectin (such as corn starch as opposed to rice) might be preferable for the infant.

FAT DIGESTION

The ability to digest fat is especially important during the neonatal period because the rapid growth rate requires an abundant supply of energy and nutrients (including fat-soluble vitamins), and because lipids are essential in the development of the central nervous system. Although the fat content of milk varies among species, it always constitutes a major proportion of the total energy. Human milk, for instance, contains 35–45 g fat per litre (see Fig. 4.1), supplying 40–50% of the total energy (Dieu and Lentner, 1970). Absorption of fat is very efficient in children and adults, but the absence of pancreatic lipase and the reduced secretion of bile salts in the newborn have raised questions as to the adequacy of the digestion of fat during the neonatal period.

The importance of gastric lipolysis was recognized recently when it was shown that lipase activity in the stomach was not due simply to contamination from pancreatic secretions but also to lingual lipase (Lebenthal, 1981; Hamosh *et al.* 1985), an enzyme derived from the serosal secretion of the Von Ebner's gland located on the posterior area of the tongue. The low optimum pH of lingual lipase is particularly well suited for the acidic environment of the stomach. In addition, a lipase secreted by the gastric mucosa has been identified. Lingual and gastric lipases cannot hydrolyse phospholipids and cholesterol, but partly hydrolyse triacylglycerols to produce a mixture of monoacylglycerols, diacylglycerols and free fatty acids (Fig. 4.11). Gastric lipase is able to hydrolyse long-chain triacylglycerols, whereas lingual lipase is restricted to medium-chain and short-chain triacylglycerols. Pancreatic lipase and its cofactor colipase are secreted into the duodenal lumen and complete the lipolysis initiated by lingual and gastric lipolysis. Pancreatic lipase hydrolyses long-chain triacylglycerols, phospholipids and cholesterol esters.

Luminal digestion of lipids is followed by the formation of micelles containing the insoluble products of lipolysis to facilitate their diffusion through the unstirred water layer that is a diffusion barrier between the intestinal lumen and the microvillous membrane (Fig. 4.12). Bile salts act as biological detergents to form small molecular aggregates with water-insoluble products of lipolysis: free fatty acids, monoacylglycerols, hydrolysed phospholipids and cholesterol. Micelles containing bile salts diffuse through the unstirred layer faster than do fatty acids in monomolecular solution. The translocation through the membrane of the brush border is thought to be due to passive diffusion under pressure of a steep gradient of concentration. Micelles break apart in the immediate vicinity of the membrane as a consequence of the protonation of the fatty acids in the acidic microenvironment. Because of their hydrophobicity, fatty acids diffuse easily through the lipid bilayer of the membrane. In the cytoplasm of the enterocyte, fatty acid and cholesterol are transported to the endoplasmic reticulum by fatty acid-binding proteins and sterol-binding proteins respectively. In the reticulum, fatty acids are once again esterified into triacylglycerols, phospholipids and cholesterol esters and are assembled with apoproteins to form prechylomicrons. The core of the aggregate contains mostly triacylglycerols, while cholesterol phospholipids and proteins are on the surface. These lipoprotein globules are then glycosylated in the Golgi and wrapped in Golgi vesicles. Vesicles fuse with the basolateral membrane of the enterocyte in a process known as exocytosis and the chylomicrons are released in the extracellular space. The chylomicrons

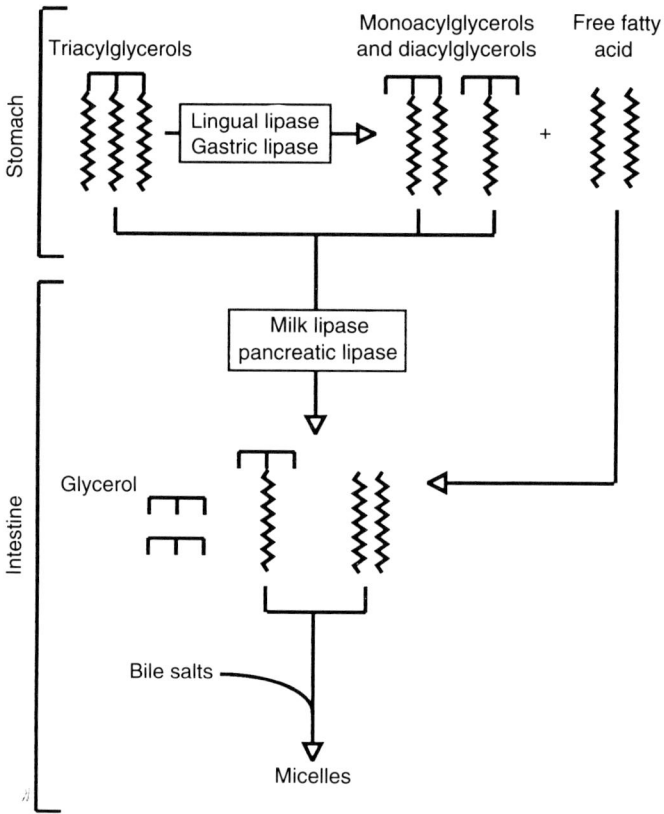

Figure 4.11 Luminal digestion of fat.

then diffuse through the basement membrane and reach the lymphatic vessels.

Our knowledge of the development of the various components of lipid absorption during the perinatal period in the human is still incomplete, making it difficult to evaluate the capacity of the newborn to handle dietary fat. One month after birth, pancreatic lipase is barely detectable in the duodenum, but at 2 years of age activity of the enzyme is equal to that in the adult (Grand *et al.* 1976; Lebenthal, 1981; Hamosh *et al.* 1985; Henning, 1987). In the rat, pancreatic lipase appears during the third week after birth and is fully active by the end of the weaning (Grand *et al.* 1976; Henning, 1987). Although human infants and especially pre-terms do not absorb fat as completely as adults, milk triacylglycerols are usually well tolerated. The current view is that preduodenal lipolysis by lingual lipase and gastric lipase may play a more important role in infants than in

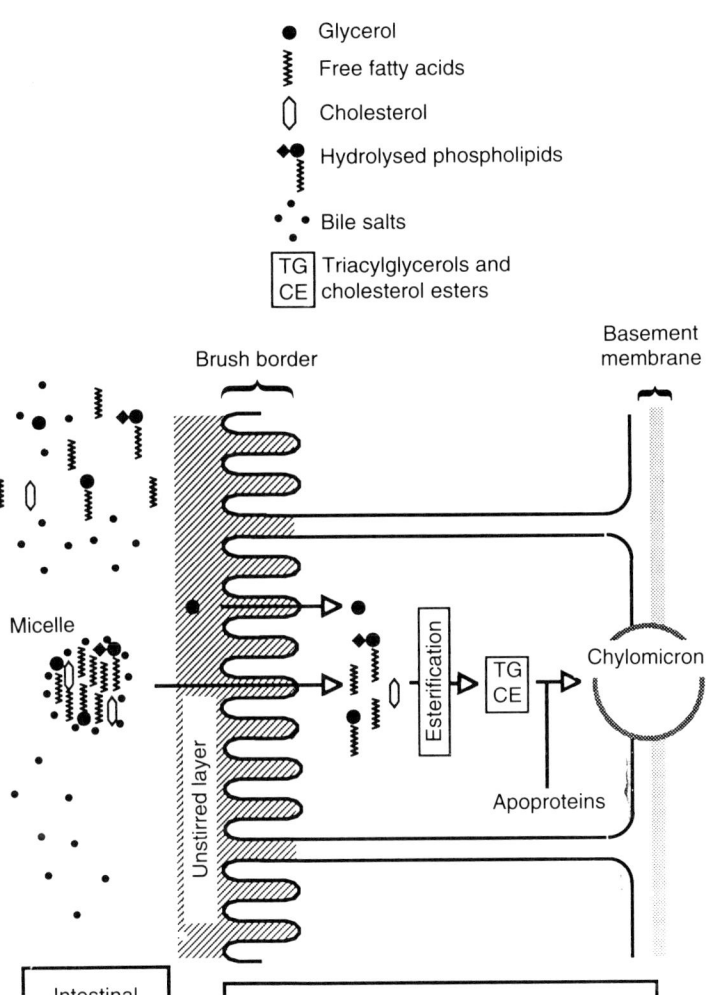

● Glycerol

Free fatty acids

Cholesterol

Hydrolysed phospholipids

Bile salts

TG Triacylglycerols and
CE cholesterol esters

Figure 4.12 Mucosal absorption of lipids.

adults (Hamosh *et al.* 1985; Henning, 1987). Lingual lipase was found in gastric aspirates of pre-terms as early as 26 weeks of gestational age. In full-term infants, activity of this enzyme is comparable to that of the adult and the relatively moderate acidity of the gastric contents is well suited to the low optimum pH of the enzyme. Milk fat is found in the form of globules with triacylglycerols in the core and phospholipids, cholesterol and protein forming a membrane as in chylomicrons (Fig. 4.13). Milk fat

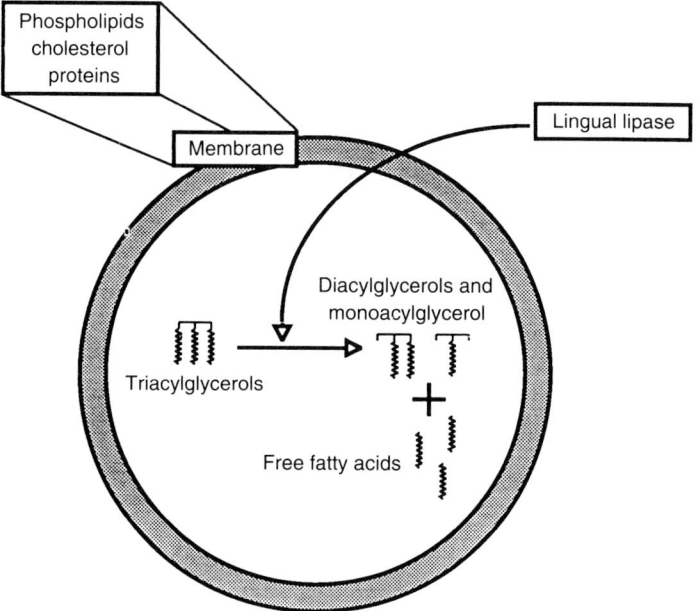

Figure 4.13 The milk fat globule.

globules are resistant to hydrolysis by pancreatic lipase, but lingual lipase can penetrate the membrane and hydrolyse the triacylglycerols in the core. Intestinal lipolysis by pancreatic lipase is facilitated by prior gastric lipolysis and possibly by hydrolysis of glycosyl-ceramides by phlorizin hydrolase.

Newborns generally utilize the fat from human milk more efficiently than the fat from cows' milk or formulas. This observation remained a subject of speculation until it was found that milk from humans and other primates has a unique characteristic of containing a lipase in an inactive form (Hernell and Blackberg, 1982). Activation requires the presence of bile salts. This enzyme is resistant to peptic proteolysis and thus reaches the duodenum intact. Bile salt-activated lipase is heat-labile, and activity is destroyed by boiling or pasteurization. An interesting difference between bile salt-activated lipase and pancreatic lipase is that the former hydrolyses triacylglycerols completely to glycerol and three free fatty acids. These products of lipolysis are less hydrophobic and can therefore be absorbed more easily than the monoacylglycerol product of pancreatic lipase, especially with the relatively low bile salt concentrations found in the new-born intestine. Thus it appears that although the digestive system of the human infant has not yet fully developed its own lipolytic system, the fat from maternal milk is efficiently absorbed. The limited capacity for absorption of fat from other sources, particularly the long-chain triacylglycerols that are poorly hydrolysed by lingual lipase, should be considered in the preparation of formulas prepared for infants and particularly for pre-terms.

LACTOSE INTOLERANCE

The postnatal evolution of lactase activity varies importantly among individuals of particular ethnic groups, and the typical patterns also vary between populations (Kretchmer, 1981). Worldwide the dominant pattern is a progressive decline of lactase activity throughout infancy and childhood, resulting in an adult specific activity of one-tenth that of the newborn. Lactose intolerance is a general term referring to the inability of an individual to efficiently digest and absorb lactose, with the resultant typical symptoms of malabsorption following ingestion of milk or a lactose-containing food. The symptoms are abdominal distention, intestinal cramps, flatulence, diarrhoea and vomiting. Persistence of acute malabsorption is of great clinical concern since it could result in dehydration and reduced absorption of nutrients. Diarrhoea can cause damage to the intestinal mucosa. In most cases of malabsorption, the symptoms disappear when lactose is removed from the diet. At this point it is important to make a distinction between two different types of lactose intolerance: the complete absence of lactase activity at birth versus the dramatically reduced activity in adults who had normal lactase activity during their childhood. A rare condition has been observed in a few individuals who were born without an enzymically active lactase. This is thought to be the manifestation of a genetic defect consisting of a mutation of the gene coding for lactase. Similar enzymic deficiencies have been found with other intestinal digestive enzymes: sucrase–isomaltase or trehalase for instance. These lactase-deficient infants were given formulas containing glucose or sucrose as the main carbohydrate with no further complications, but will have to avoid ingesting lactose throughout life. This condition is distinct from that of infants born prematurely who do not have a sufficient activity of lactase to completely digest lactose in maternal milk and might have similar signs of malabsorption. Pre-term infants usually develop normal lactase activity rapidly after birth and can be breast fed thereafter.

The progressive decline of lactase activity in humans is similar to the decline of activity observed in animal models such as rats or rabbits and is considered to be the normal pattern of expression of lactase activity. Several mechanisms have been suggested (Subcommittee on the Evaluation of the Safety of Modified Starches in Infant Foods, 1977;

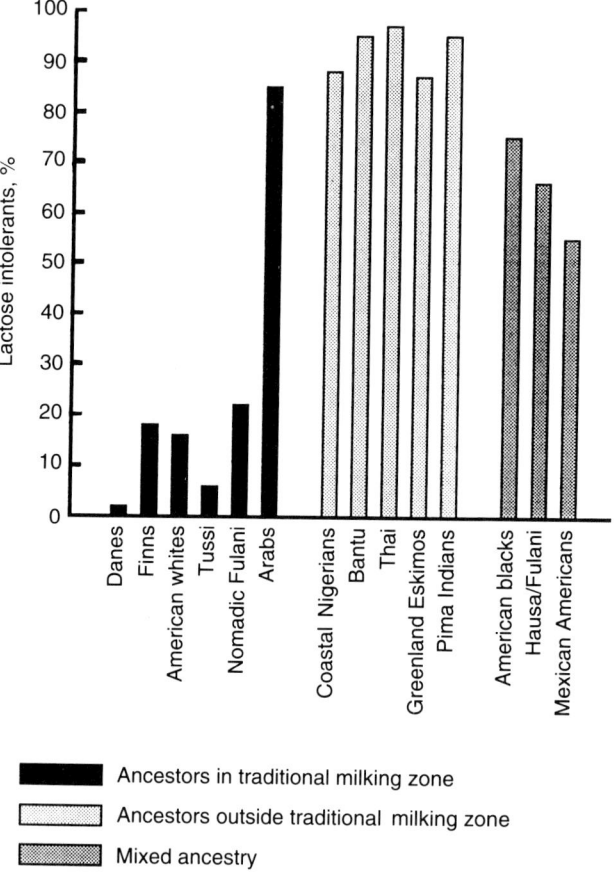

Figure 4.14 Distribution of lactose intolerance in adults in different populations. (Data from Kretchmer, 1981.)

Kretchmer, 1981; Mobassaleh *et al.* 1985) to explain this decline, including a faster cellular turnover in the adult epithelium that would not allow for accumulation of as much enzyme, a reduced rate of synthesis, or an increase in the rate of degradation. The details of the mechanism responsible for the decline of lactase activity remain to be ascertained but it is clear that it is a genetically programmed series of events (Kretchmer, 1981). The persistence of an elevated lactase activity in adulthood is seen as a failure of that decline to take place. Individuals with high lactase activity are found in all human populations but in proportions that seem to indicate a situation in which food would have been the selective agent (Kretchmer, 1981). The majority of adults are lactose-intolerant except in

Northwestern Europeans and some African and Indian populations that are descended from ancestors known to have raised livestock and to whom dairy products were available (Fig. 4.14). Even though daily consumption of fresh milk by the adults of these ancient populations is not well documented, the ability to digest dairy products occasionally when other sources of food were scarce could have been a strong evolutionary advantage. Any mutation that impaired the mechanism responsible for the normal decline of lactase and the subsequent inability to digest milk would thus be preserved and encountered with a higher prevalence in those particular populations.

REFERENCES

Auricchio, S., Stellato, A. and de Vizia, B. (1981) Development of brush border peptidases in human and rat small intestine during fetal and neonatal life. *Pediatric Research*, **15**, 991–995.

Crane, R.K. (1975) The physiology of the intestinal absorption of sugars. In *Physiological Effects of Food Carbohydrates*, pp. 2–19 (ed J.A. Hodges). Washington, DC: American Chemical Society.

Deren, J.S. (1971) Development of structure and function in the fetal and newborn stomach. *American Journal of Clinical Nutrition*, **24**, 144–159.

Dieu, C. and Lentner, C. (eds) (1970) *Scientific Tables*, 7th edn, pp. 688–689. Basel: Ciba-Geigy.

Doell, R. and Kretchmer, N. (1962) Studies of the small intestine during development. I. Distribution and activity of β-galactosidase. *Biochimica et Biophysica Acta*, **62**, 353–362.

Dymsza, H.A., Czajka, D.M. and Miller, S.A. (1964) Influence of artificial diet on weight gain and body composition of the neonatal rat. *Journal of Nutrition*, **84**, 100–106.

Gracey, M., Burke, V. and Oshin, A. (1970) Intestinal transport of fructose. *Lancet*, **ii**, 827–828.

Grand, R.J., Watkins, J.B. and Torti, F.M. (1976) Development of the human gastrointestinal tract. *Gastroenterology*, **70**, 790–810.

Hadorn, B. (1981) Developmental aspects of intraluminal protein digestion. In *Textbook of Gastroenterology and Nutrition in Infancy*, vol. 1. *Gastrointestinal Development and Perinatal Nutrition*, pp. 365–373. (ed. E. Lebenthal). New York: Raven Press.

Hamosh, M., Bitman, J., Wood, D.L. *et al.* (1985) Lipids in milk and the first steps in their digestion. *Pediatrics*, **75** (Suppl.), 146–150.

Henning, S. (1981) Postnatal development: coordination of feeding, digestion, and metabolism. *American Journal of Physiology*, **241**, G199–G214.

Henning, S.J. (1985) Ontogeny of enzymes of the small intestine. *Annual Reviews of Physiology*, **47**, 231–245.

Henning, S.J. (1987) Functional development of the gastrointestinal tract. In *Physiology of the Gastrointestinal Tract*, pp. 285–300 (ed. L.R. Johnson). New York: Raven Press.

Henning, S. and Kretchmer, N. (1973) Development of intestinal function in mammals. *Enzyme*, **15**, 3–23.

Henning, S.J., Chang, S.S.P. and Gisel, E.G. (1979) Ontogeny of feeding controls in suckling and weanling rats. *American Journal of Physiology*, 237, R187–R191.

Hernell, O. and Blackberg, L. (1982) Digestion of human milk lipids: physiologic significance of *sn-*2 monoacylglycerol hydrolysis by bile salt stimulated lipase. *Pediatric Research*, 16, 882–885.

Klein, R. and McKenzie, J.C. (1983) The role of cell renewal in the ontogeny of the intestine. I. Cell proliferation patterns in adult, fetal, and neonatal intestine. *Journal of Pediatric Gastroenterology and Nutrition*, 2, 10–43.

Kretchmer, N. (1981) Food: a selective agent in evolution. In *Food Nutrition and Evolution*, pp. 37–48 (eds D.N. Walcher and N. Kretchmer). New York: Masson.

Kretchmer, N. (1985) Weaning: enzymatic adaptation. *American Journal of Clinical Nutrition*, 41, 391–398.

Lebenthal, E. (1981) *Textbook of Gastroenterology and Nutrition in Infancy*, vol. 1. *Gastrointestinal Development and Perinatal Nutrition*. New York: Raven Press.

Lebenthal, E. (1989) *Human Gastrointestinal Development*. New York: Raven Press.

Mobassaleh, M., Montgomery, R.K., Biller, J.A. and Grand, R.J. (1985) Development of carbohydrate absorption in the fetus and neonate. *Pediatrics*, 75, 160–166.

Raul, F., Lacroix, B. and Aprahamian, M. (1986) Longitudinal distribution of brush border hydrolases and morphological maturation in the intestine of the preterm infant. *Early Human Development*, 13, 225–234.

Semenza, G. (1986) Anchoring and biosynthesis of stalked brush border membrane proteins. *Annual Review of Cell Biology*, 2, 255–313.

Sigrist-Nelson, K. and Hopfer, U. (1974) A distinct D-fructose transport system in isolated brush-border membrane. *Biochimica et Biophysica Acta*, 367, 247–254.

Subcommittee on the Evaluation of the Safety of Modified Starches in Infant Foods: Committee on Nutrition (1977) *Safety and Suitability of Modified Food Starches for Use in Baby Food*. Houston: American Academy of Pediatrics.

Sunshine, P., Herbst, J.J., Koldovsky, O. and Kretchmer, N. (1971) Adaption of the gastrointestinal tract to extrauterine life. *Annals of the New York Academy of Science*, 176, 16–29.

Taylor, W.H. (1968) Biochemistry of pepsins. In *Handbook of Physiology*, section 6, vol. 5, pp. 2567–2587 (ed. C.F. Code). Washington, DC: American Physiological Society.

Walker, W.A. (1985) Absorption of protein and protein fragments in the developing intestine: role in immunologic/allergic reactions. *Pediatrics*, 75, 167–171.

Younoszai, M.K. (1974) Jejunal absorption of hexose in infants and adults. *Journal of Pediatrics*, 85, 446–448.

5
Infant growth and energy requirements: updating reference values

Alison A. Paul, Peter S.W. Davies and
Roger G. Whitehead
MRC Dunn Nutrition Centre, Cambridge, UK

INTRODUCTION

In common with all primates, the human infant is characterized by a relatively slow growth rate in comparison with other mammalian species. A greater proportion of dietary energy is therefore used for maintenance requirements and a smaller amount for growth. In spite of this, there is no doubt that differences in growth are found according to mode of feeding. Secular changes in breast feeding and timing and amounts of solid foods have resulted in changing patterns of weight gain and the laying down of subcutaneous fat. Present-day infants grow less rapidly and are thinner than those who comprised growth standards drawn up a generation or more ago. Should these standards now be revised to reflect current feeding practices? Does a lowered energy intake indicate a lower energy requirement, or have previous dietary recommendations been set too high?

TRENDS IN INFANT FEEDING

Breast and bottle feeding

The majority of infants in Britain today are bottle-fed by the age of 6 weeks. This is despite official advice from the Department of Health that

Infant Nutrition. Edited by A.F. Walker and B.A. Rolls.
Published in 1994 by Chapman & Hall, London.
ISBN 0 412 59140 5.

all mothers should be encouraged to breast feed their babies (DHSS, 1988). In 1985, 64% of mothers started to breast feed, but by 6 weeks post partum only 38% were still doing so, falling to 21% by 6 months (Martin and White, 1988). Before the 1950s, breast feeding was more common, but over the next two decades a more rapid decline set in, as shown in Fig. 5.1 (Whitehead and Paul, 1987). A nadir was reached in the early 1970s, when only 24% of mothers in England were breast feeding at 3 months. This alerted health professionals to give more encouragement to breast feeding, with the result that there was a welcome return to this mode of feeding up to the early 1980s. A plateau now seems to have been reached, with little further change between 1980 and 1985.

Concurrent with the secular increase in the numbers of babies who were bottle-fed, there have been profound changes in the composition of formula milks, and in the way mothers are instructed to make up bottles. In earlier times, bottle feeds consisted of diluted cows' milk plus extra sugar to bring the composition of the energy-providing constituents approximately to that of breast milk. Full cream powdered infant milks

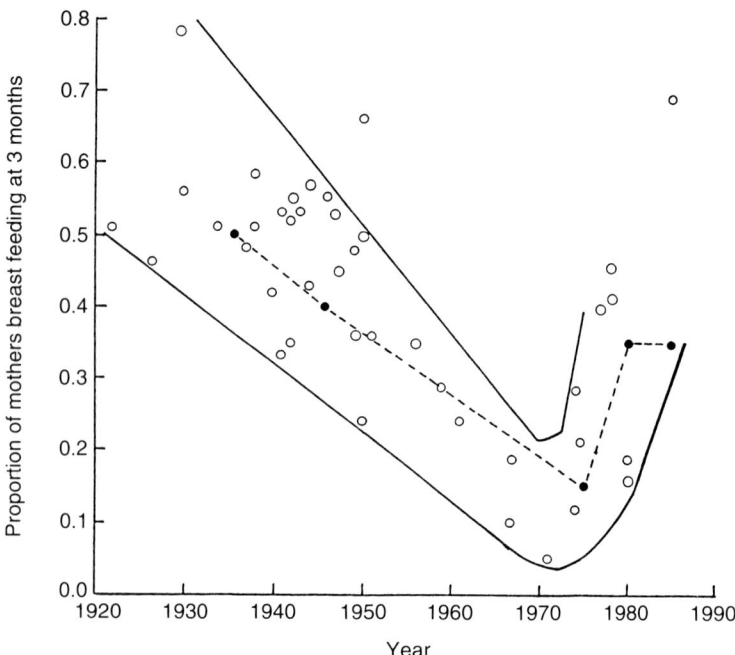

Figure 5.1 Proportions of mothers breast feeding at 3 months in England and Wales from 1920 to 1985: (●) national surveys; (○) individual cities and towns from 29 different studies (Whitehead and Paul, 1987).

also required sugar to be added during the feed preparation. These practices gave more scope for error, and the tendency to ensure that the baby was getting enough food meant that feeds were also often over-concentrated. Concern about the prevalence of obesity in babies (Taitz, 1971), and the adverse consequences of hypernatraemia (Davies, 1973), led to modification of the formulas based on full cream cows' milk to a composition aimed to be closer to that of breast milk. By 1976, full cream milk formulas were no longer available, and only modified milks are now made, in which extra carbohydrate is incorporated. Most or all of the butterfat is replaced, usually by vegetable fats, and in some there is a higher proportion of whey to casein than is present in cows' milk.

Introduction of solids

In this respect too, there have been major changes over the past 70 years, as shown in Fig. 5.2. In the 1920s, it was customary to recommend that babies should receive nothing but milk for the first 9 months. By the 1940s, this age had been reduced to 6 months, further reducing to 3–4 months by the 1960s (Whitehead and Paul, 1987). The gap between recommendations and practice became wider as mothers were giving solids earlier and earlier, until by the mid-1970s it was not unusual to find

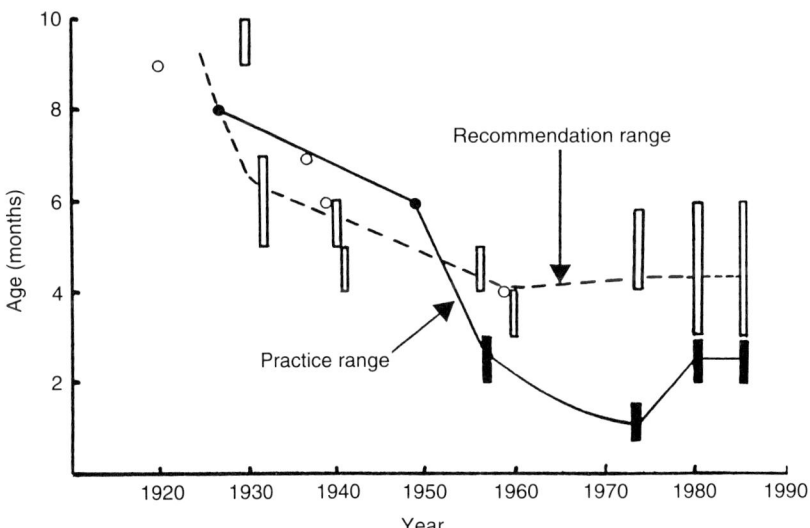

Figure 5.2 Ages of introduction of solid foods in the UK from 1920 to 1985 (Whitehead and Paul, 1987): (O– – –O) means or ranges of recommendations given by various authors advising on infant feeding; (●——●) means or ranges of reported age of introduction.

babies of only 2 weeks old being given non-milk foods (DHSS, 1974). Concern arising from such findings led to active promotion of recommendations to delay starting solids until 3–4 months, with encouraging results. The position appears to have stabilized since 1980, the most recent national figures for 1985 showing that only about 10% of babies received solids at 6 weeks of age compared with 40% in 1975. By 3 months the corresponding figures were 60% and 90% (Martin and White, 1988). As bottle-feeding mothers introduce solids earlier than those who breast feed, the national data on ages of starting solids are also influenced by the changes in proportions of mothers who are breast or bottle feeding.

GROWTH OF BREAST-FED AND BOTTLE-FED BABIES

Since bottle feeding became a widespread alternative way of rearing a baby, comparisons have been made between the growth of breast-fed and bottle-fed babies. In the early years of this century, underfeeding and failure to thrive were the common danger in bottle feeding, as it is in the Third World today, and breast-fed infants were shown to have superior weight gain (Aitken and Hytten, 1960). As hygienic practices improved, bottle feeding became less hazardous, and by the 1950s babies fed this way showed greater weight gains (Ministry of Health, 1959). By the late 1960s, with the predominance of bottle feeding, overfeeding became the problem and excessive weight gains gave cause for concern (Taitz, 1971). Over the last 20 years, with the introduction of modified milk formulas and greater attention to correct feeding practices, weight gains of bottle-fed infants are no longer excessive, but a small differential between breast- and bottle-fed infants can still be seen, as shown in Fig. 5.3 for groups of Cambridge infants. Similar findings have been reported from Australia and the USA (Hitchcock *et al.* 1985; Czajka-Narins and Jung, 1986). In the Cambridge sample, as in those from other countries, it is notable that the divergence of the weight curves did not begin until after 6 months of age, so the effect is less likely to be a consequence of the milk itself, but rather of the total dietary pattern in later infancy.

The weight differential in the Cambridge babies was to some extent due to a smaller accumulation of body fat in those who were breast-fed, as shown in Fig. 5.4 for subscapular skinfold thickness. However, triceps skinfold thickness did not show any difference between breast-fed and bottle-fed babies. Of greater relevance was that there was also no disparity in length gain according to mode of milk feeding.

The weaning period for breast-fed infants

A bigger influence on weight gain in the second half of infancy related to the timing of introducing weaning foods. This in turn was associated with

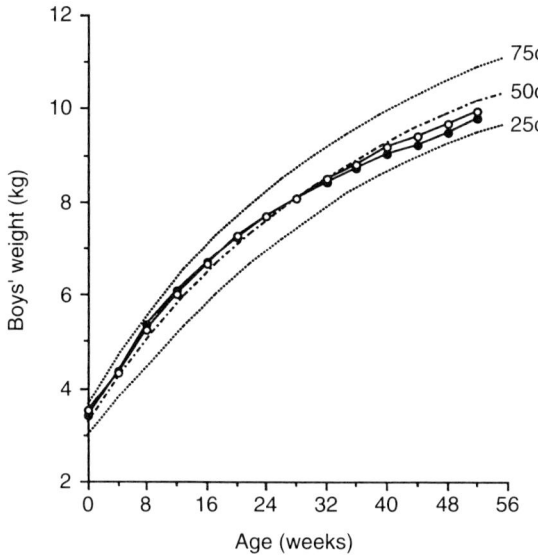

Figure 5.3 Weights in the first year of Cambridge boys breast-fed to at least 24 weeks or bottle-fed from 3 weeks or less compared with standard NCHS centiles (Hamill *et al.* 1977): (●) breast-fed, *n* = 57; (○) bottle-fed, *n* = 35.

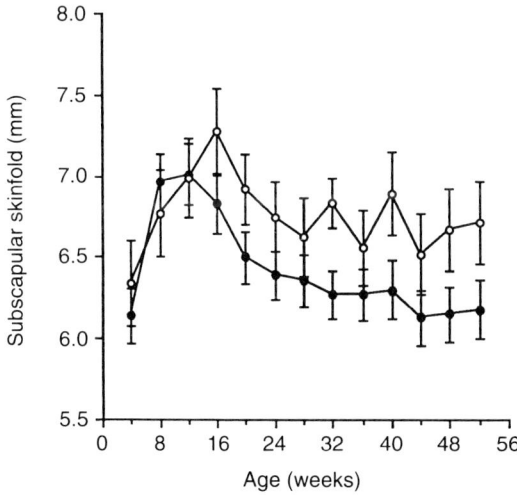

Figure 5.4 Subscapular skinfold thicknesses in the first year of Cambridge boys breast-fed to at least 24 weeks or bottle-fed from 3 weeks or less: (●) breast-fed, *n* = 56; (○) bottle-fed, *n* = 35. Values are mean and SEM.

the length of time that breast feeding itself was continued, as the mothers who introduced solids later were also those who breast fed the longest. Dividing the Cambridge breast-fed boys into those given solids before or after 16 weeks (Fig. 5.5) showed that the weight gain was slower in those not given solids at an early age, but the differences were not apparent until 9–12 months of age. Even more marked decelerations are shown in other studies of babies exclusively breast-fed until at least 6 months (Chandra, 1982; Salmenpera *et al.* 1985).

GROWTH STANDARDS FOR INFANCY

Much of the argument on the adequacy of infant feeding hinges on growth in comparison with standard patterns. The two most commonly used standards, those of Tanner in the UK (Tanner *et al.* 1966; Tanner and Whitehouse, 1975) and the National Center for Health Statistics (NCHS) in the USA (Hamill *et al.* 1977), also adopted by WHO (1978), are derived from measurements made many years ago, when infant feeding practices were different. Few of the infants who comprise the NCHS

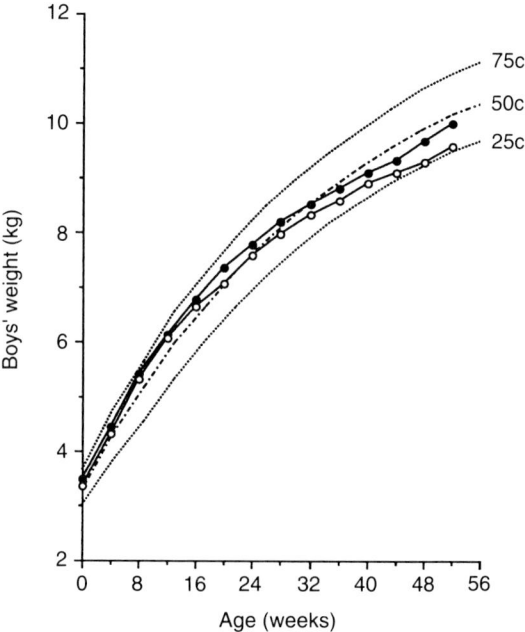

Figure 5.5 Weights in the first year of Cambridge breast-fed boys according to age of introduction of solids: (●) before 16 weeks, *n* = 28; (○) 16 weeks or later, *n* = 29. Standard NCHS centiles (Hamill *et al.* 1977) are also shown.

standards were breast-fed, and the measurements were made between 1929 and 1975. The Tanner skinfold measurements were made in 1966, only a small percentage of the infants were breast-fed, and a proportion of them were overweight (Hutchinson-Smith, 1973). The standards undoubtedly reflected feeding patterns of that period, but are inappropriate for use now.

It became apparent through studies on lactation and infant growth (Whitehead and Paul, 1984; Whitehead *et al.* 1989) that breast-fed infants who lived in good socioeconomic circumstances were showing characteristic growth patterns that differed from the standards. An initial weight gain to above the 50th centile was followed from 3–4 months by a relative deceleration in relation to the standard which did not halt until the end of the first year. Such patterns are widely reported from developing countries (Waterlow *et al.* 1980; Whitehead and Paul, 1984), where weight faltering is a serious health problem, but to see it from advantaged infants, albeit to a smaller extent, was unexpected. To investigate this further, a large-scale study was initiated in Cambridge, which confirmed and extended the findings. The widespread demonstrations in this and other studies of a deceleration in weight after about 4 months, and the markedly smaller skinfold thicknesses, call into question the appropriateness of currently available standards for present-day infants.

The Cambridge infant growth study

The Cambridge infant growth study was set up in 1983, to provide data on infant feeding and growth. Of the infants in the study, 90% were initially breast-fed, 69% were still being so fed at 12 weeks and 58% at 24 weeks; 6% were receiving solids by 8 weeks, 38% by 12 weeks and 74% by 16 weeks. A high proportion therefore were fed in accordance with the advice from the DHSS (1988). Of the families studied, 58% belonged to the non-manual social classes (I, II and III NM), a proportion broadly representative of Cambridge.

The anthropometric results have been prepared in centile form, and are given in Figs 5.6–5.9. These interim results are derived from the first two cohorts that were recruited, but they are essentially the same when all four cohorts (which comprise the whole study) are considered together. Smoothed centiles have been prepared for the first year of life (Whitehead *et al.* 1989), using the recently developed LMS method of Cole (1988). This is a procedure that summarizes the data by three smooth curves which represent the median, coefficient of variation and skewness of the variable's distribution as it changes with age.

Weight and length were compared with the NCHS standards (Hamill *et al.* 1977), but very similar patterns were shown if the Tanner standards

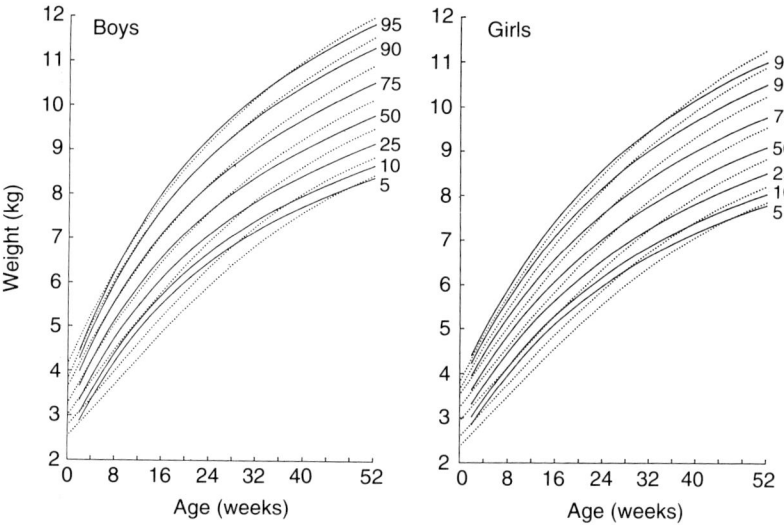

Figure 5.6 Fifth to ninety-fifth centiles of weights in the first year of Cambridge babies (72 boys and 60 girls) (———) compared with NCHS standard centiles (Hamill *et al.* 1977) (· · · ·).

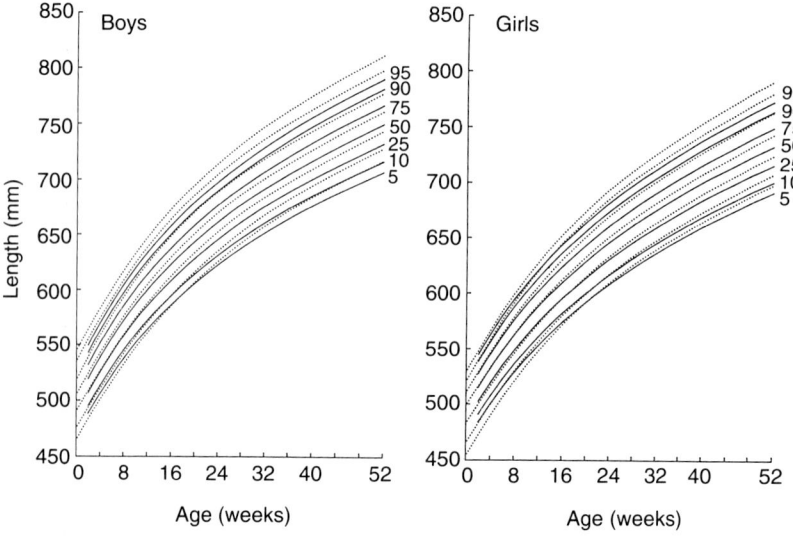

Figure 5.7 Fifth to ninety-fifth centiles of recumbent lengths in the first year of Cambridge babies (72 boys and 60 girls) (———) compared with NCHS standard centiles (Hamill *et al.* 1977) (· · · ·).

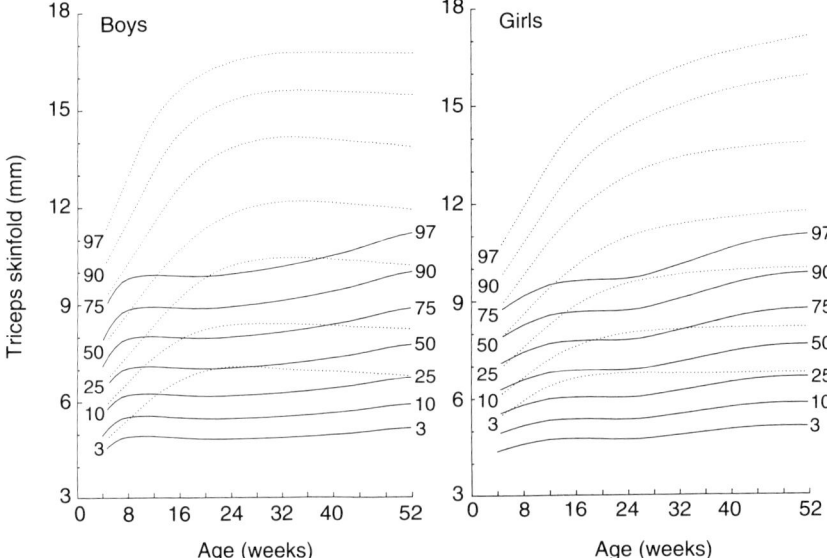

Figure 5.8 Third to ninety-seventh centiles of triceps skinfold thicknesses in the first year of Cambridge babies (72 boys and 60 girls) (———) compared with Tanner and Whitehouse (1975) standard centiles (· · · ·).

(Tanner *et al.* 1966) were used instead (Whitehead *et al.* 1988). Tanner skinfold standards, which were revised in 1975 (Tanner and Whitehouse, 1975), are also shown in Figs 5.8 and 5.9.

In both boys and girls, the Cambridge weight centiles confirmed the earlier indications of a pattern different from the standards, with an acceleration over the first 4 months, followed by a slower weight gain to the end of the first year. It was not confined to breast-fed infants, as can be seen in Fig. 5.3. Length also showed a deficit by 1 year, although the initial spurt was not present. The most pronounced differences were found with skinfold thicknesses, triceps in particular showing the striking absence of the rapid fat accumulation illustrated in the standards over the first 6 months. The Cambridge 50th centile was below the Tanner 10th centile for the whole of the first year. Subscapular skinfold was also reduced in the Cambridge infants, their 50th centile corresponding only to Tanner's 10–25th centiles. Again, this was regardless of whether the infants were breast- or bottle-fed (see Fig. 5.4). Very similar values were found by Schluter *et al.* (1976) in Germany and Yeung (1983) in Canada, their 50th centiles being more akin to Tanner's original standards of the 1950s (Tanner and Whitehouse, 1962).

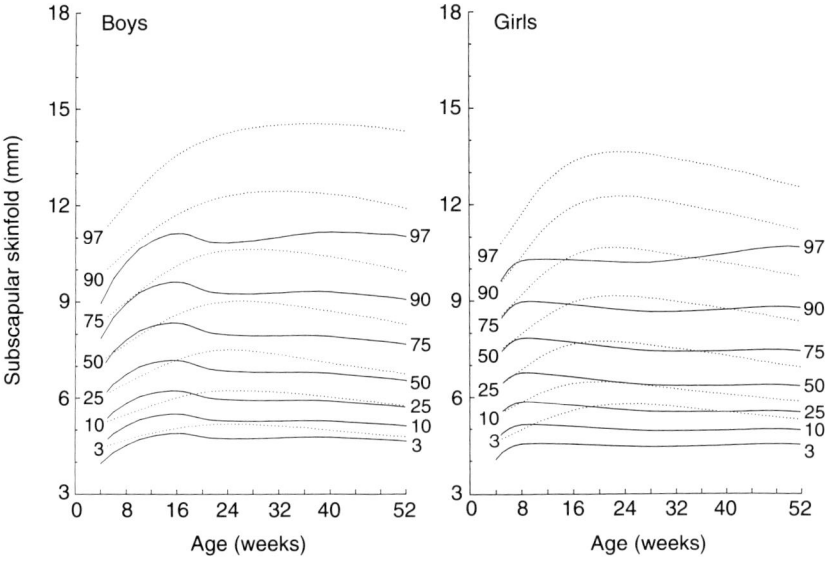

Figure 5.9 Third to ninety-seventh centiles of subscapular skinfold thicknesses in the first year of Cambridge babies (72 boys and 60 girls) (———) compared with Tanner and Whitehouse (1975) standard centiles (· · · ·).

Is there a need for new growth standards for infancy?

Growth standards for infancy have not received as much attention as those for later ages, particularly adolescence, which have been extensively studied. Of special relevance for current weight and length standards for infancy is that measurements were made at too infrequent intervals to reflect accurately the rapid changes that occur during the first year of life. Monthly velocities obtained by interpolation over 3-monthly intervals cannot take sufficient account of the very rapid growth, particularly in the first 2 months, even though the NCHS standard does include a measurement at 1 month of age. In contrast, the Cambridge data were obtained from measurements made every 4 weeks throughout the first year. That the apparently different growth pattern is partly statistical in origin is well illustrated by examination of the new monthly reference values prepared by Roche *et al.* (1989) from some of the data in the Fels longitudinal study that were used for the NCHS standards. A spurt in weight gain over the first few months, followed by a subsequent decline, is clearly seen when the new monthly reference data are compared with the NCHS standards (see Fig. 5.10). Comparison of the Cambridge data with the new Roche values removes some of the relative decline in weight in later

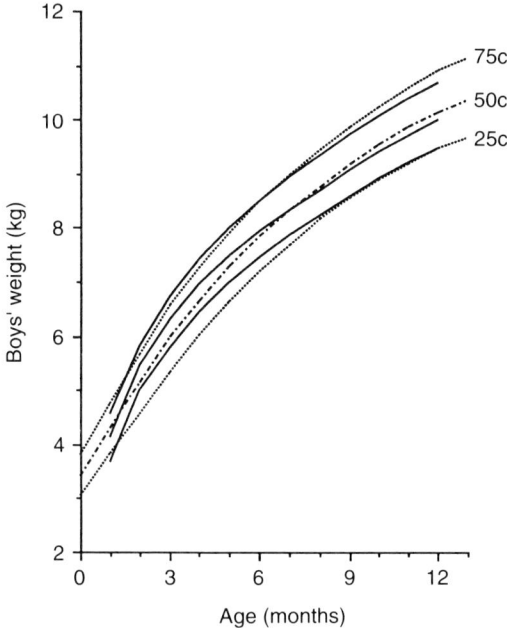

Figure 5.10 Monthly reference values for weight from 1 to 12 months of age (Roche *et al.* 1989) (———) compared with NCHS standard centiles (Hamill *et al.* 1977) (· · · ·).

infancy, but it is still present. However, the original NCHS/Child Development Center (CDC) centiles are widely used, and since being adopted by the WHO for their international charts (WHO, 1978) provide a yardstick by which nutritional assessments can be compared within and between all countries (Sullivan *et al.* 1991). They also have the advantage of having computer software available for the calculation of standard deviation scores (*Z* scores) and percentiles, which are being increasingly used in presentation of growth data. There are arguments for and against having separate standards for babies according to the way they are fed, or indeed for different countries, environments or disease states. While it would be impractical to construct standards to cater for every situation, the aim should be to have up-to-date standards reflecting overall current feeding practices. A country's standards can change over the years. In Australia, for example, the 1960s weight standard was higher than the 1930s, but recent measurements have reverted to nearer those of the 1930s (Gracey, 1987). The Netherlands standards also showed reduction in weight at 1 year between 1965 and 1980 (Roede and van Wieringen, 1985). The UK growth standards are currently under review, as new data are available both for infants and children. In the meantime, knowledge of growth expectations in definable groups, e.g. breast-fed infants, should be used alongside any existing standards.

Practical importance of growth differences

Standard infant growth charts, especially for weight, are used to assess the adequacy of breast feeding and weaning practices. The basic assumption is that while the growth of a child runs parallel to the appropriate centile lines then all is well, but when it starts to cross centile lines downwards then all is not well. It is becoming increasingly recognized that breast-fed infants in particular grow more slowly than currently available standards, and that this should be accepted as their normal growth pattern. There do not appear to be deleterious consequences with respect to health and physical activity associated with this lower growth velocity (Dewey *et al.* 1990). Comparing an *individual* breast-fed baby against a group of breast-fed babies rather than the standard will provide a different interpretation of its growth performance. The age at which growth might be considered unsatisfactory could differ by 2 or 3 months. This is of considerable relevance to the giving of advice on introducing solids in Third World countries. The later this can be delayed without compromising the child's growth the better, because of the risks of contamination of weaning foods with microorganisms.

The apparent weight deficit of normal breast-fed babies in relation to standards is also relevant in the UK with respect to concern about the 'sudden infant death syndrome' (SIDS) and the effective monitoring of the child who is likely to be at risk. One way that has been suggested is via frequent weighing of the child and the careful plotting of growth charts. If the child shows *marked* downward crossing of more than two channel widths in 8 weeks on specially constructed Sheffield charts, he or she is considered to be in need of special surveillance (Emery *et al.* 1985). The degree of growth retardation in the truly at-risk SIDS case is, of course, greater than we have described for the Cambridge breast-fed babies. However, this does emphasize the importance that is being attached to the shape of centile lines and the consequent need to ensure that they are correct if mothers and health workers are not to be worried unnecessarily.

Long-term significances of infant growth

Our investigations plus those of other workers currently studying child growth are clearly showing that growth parameters of even healthy children are very sensitive to changes in dietary pattern. Inevitably the question arises as to the long-term significance. So far, our first cohorts have reached only 5–6 years of age, but their results are similar to those in a previous study up to 7 years (Paul *et al.* 1990). Although it is premature to make any definitive comments, the data indicate that the downward crossing of the weight and length centiles did not halt until the middle of the second year. After that, some increase in growth was seen. Whether it matters to have had a slight deficit at a particular stage in infancy cannot readily be determined, but if such children do not eventually catch up it will contrast with other findings where increased height has been shown in children in recent years, for example by Chinn and Rona (1984).

Whether the Cambridge infants, a high proportion of whom were breast-fed, are destined to remain slightly smaller through childhood is a subject for further study, but they might be expected to become taller, rather than smaller, in view of their higher social class. Birkbeck *et al.* 1985) showed that previously breast-fed children were taller at 7 years than their bottle-fed counterparts, but they attributed this to the influence of maternal stature, which in turn was related to the more affluent socio-economic circumstances of the family rather than breast feeding itself. Studies have indicated that breast feeding provides a significant protective effect against subsequent obesity in childhood (Kramer *et al.* 1985; Hamosh, 1988). However, others have not found that weight gain in childhood was related to breast or bottle feeding in infancy (Pomerance, 1987). Clearly there are many confounding variables, and there is no consensus on whether childhood height and weight is influenced by the milk feeding *per se* in normal full-term infants.

The importance of laying down fat stores in infancy has a number of implications. It was feared at one time that fatness in infancy posed a considerably greater risk for later obesity, but this was somewhat allayed by demonstrations that most fat infants did not become fat children (Poskitt and Cole, 1977). On the other hand, most fat children were fat in infancy, so fat accumulation is an undesirable component of infant physiology in present-day countries with good standards of health care. But it may be that it is natural for the human infant to lay down a fat store in the early months, which could be used to overcome the hazards of adapting to a mixed diet over the weaning period. Certainly such situations are normal in Third World countries. Here the life-supporting release of energy from the subcutaneous fat stores during episodes of periodic infection is of great practical importance. The loss of 100 g adipose tissue would provide approximately 3 MJ (700 kcal), enough to cover the maintenance needs of a 1-year-old baby for a whole day. If lean tissue had to be used, the weight loss would be approximately 700 g. This is one reason for the dramatic weight loss of underweight children during infections: they lack adequate fat stores. It is understandable therefore that some authorities caution against dietary recommendations that might limit the capacity of the child to store fat.

ENERGY REQUIREMENTS DURING INFANCY

Components of energy expenditure and energy intake

The human neonate requires food energy for numerous and varied
biological functions. The major components of energy intake and energy
expenditure are shown in Fig. 5.11.

The energy content of food eaten by the infant can be measured using
bomb calorimetry. Samples of the ingested food are completely oxidized
in a small chamber and the energy produced by the oxidation is
calculated. This method gives rise to a calculation of *gross energy intake*.
However, not all ingested food energy is available to the infant and some
energy is inevitably lost in the urine and faeces. Thus the *metabolizable
energy intake* is the gross energy intake minus *energy lost*. A reasonable

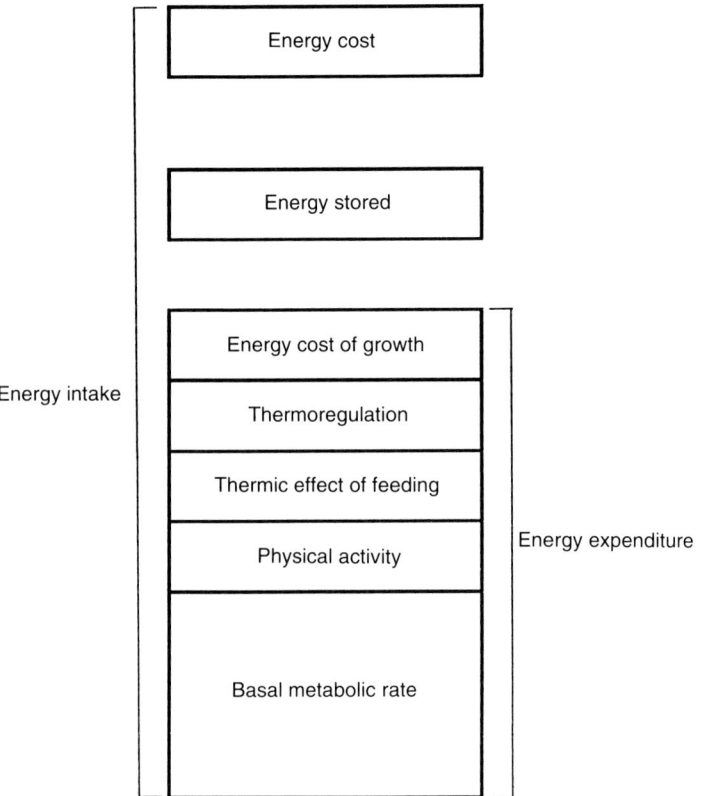

Figure 5.11 The components of total energy intake and expenditure during
infancy.

estimate of energy losses in the stool and urine is 21 kJ (5 kcal)/kg body weight per day.

The largest portion of metabolizable energy intake is expended owing to the energy cost of basic life functions, e.g. pumping ions out of cells, maintaining the heart beating, breathing, etc. Thus basal metabolic rate (BMR) is by far the largest component of total energy expenditure. The definition of a measurement of BMR makes it virtually impossible to achieve with infant subjects. The measurement requires that the subject be in a fasted state, in a thermoneutral environment, awake and not moving. The difficulty of obtaining such cooperation from infants is self-evident! Nevertheless it is relatively easy to measure *sleeping metabolic rate* in an infant. This can be achieved using indirect calorimetry. Such measurements (Schofield *et al.* 1985; P.S.W. Davies and C. Joughin, personal communication) would indicate that sleeping metabolic rate is remarkably constant and consistent in the first year of life, at about 210 kJ (50 kcal)/kg body weight per day. This is about twice the BMR of an adult (on a per kilogram body weight basis). The much larger energy requirement, per unit body weight, for basal functions in the infant is due to differences in the proportions of organs between infants and adults. The major organs responsible for large amounts of expended energy, namely the brain, heart, liver and kidneys, are a much larger proportion of total body weight in an infant, while muscle mass, which requires less basal energy expenditure, is a much higher proportion in an adult.

Sleeping metabolic rate is also influenced by the level of body fatness. Fat mass is much less metabolically active than fat-free mass and therefore very thin (e.g. small for dates) infants often have a high sleeping metabolic rate on a per kilogram body weight basis.

Thermoregulation is a further component of total energy expenditure. In normal-weight infants in the Western world the energy cost of thermoregulation is small.

The *energy cost of growth* can be divided into two parts: the energy laid down in new tissue, and the energy cost of laying down that tissue. The latter component is related to the *thermic effect of feeding*. Following a feed, the energy expended by an infant can be shown to be increased. Part of this increase is the thermic effect of feeding and is due to the energy cost of digestion and the transport of nutrients throughout the body, while some of the increased energy expenditure is undoubtedly due to the energy cost of converting digested food energy into new tissue. This growth in infancy probably occurs as discrete 'bursts' following food. The fact that sleeping metabolic rate remains the same (about 210 kJ (50 kcal)/kg per day) during the first year of life, while growth rate slows down dramatically, provides further evidence that growth is *not* a part of sleeping metabolic rate but a discrete postprandial energy cost.

The energy laid down in new tissue can be estimated if one knows growth rate and the composition of the new tissue. Using reference data (Fomon *et al.* 1982), energy stored in new tissue can be estimated and expressed as a percentage of energy intake. Such data for the first year of life are shown in Table 5.1.

The final component of total energy expenditure is that expended during *physical activity*. Until recently there have been few data available. Thus experts were forced to speculate, e.g. Waterlow (1988): 'As a guess since there is no hard information, and by analogy with adults, we might take the cost of activity at 3 months of age to be 20% greater than BMR for 12 out of 24 hours and at 6 months as 40% greater than BMR for 12 hours in the day'. A relatively new approach has been to consider the energy cost of activity as being the difference between sleeping metabolic rate and total energy expenditure (Davies, 1991). Difficulties arise, however, in the assessment of total energy expenditure in infancy. Classical methods of assessing total energy expenditure such as using direct calorimetry or heart rate monitoring are not possible in infants for ethical and practical reasons. However, the advent and subsequent development of the doubly labelled water technique for the non-invasive estimation of carbon dioxide production rate have ameliorated the situation. This technique will be described in detail later. Thus a number of studies have combined measures of total energy expenditure and sleeping metabolic rate to assess the energy cost of activity. The total energy expenditure : sleeping metabolic rate ratio (TEE : SMR) is also used as an index of activity in this context. Some of the resulting data are shown in Table 5.2.

The apparent reduction at 4 months of age of energy expended per kilogram per day on activity may be a function of the reduced number of infants studied at this time point. This possibility is enhanced as the TEE : SMR ratio tends to increase from 1.5 months onwards.

Table 5.1 The energy laid down in new tissue and its percentage of energy intake in the first year of life

Age (months)	Energy laid down in new tissue	
	kJ/day	Percentage of energy intake
0–3	699	32
3–6	385	13
6–9	188	6
9–12	151	4

Calculated from Fomon *et al.* (1982).

Table 5.2 The energy cost of activity of the ratio of total energy expenditure (TEE) and sleeping metabolic rate (SMM) found in some recent studies on infants

Age (months)	n	Energy cost of activity kJ/kg per day	TEE:SMR ratio
1[a]	20	63	1.40
1.5[b]	49	71	1.34
3[b]	50	88	1.42
4[a]	20	67	1.50
6[b]	37	121	1.58
9[b]	22	163	1.78

[a]From Butte *et al.* (1990).
[b]From Davies *et al.* (1989); Davies and Joughin (personal communication).

Energy requirements and recommendations

For almost half a century, international and national committees have made recommendations on the food energy needs of infants and children. Such recommendations have three major uses. First, knowledge of energy requirements in infancy is vital if one is to derive the special energy needs of sick children. Second, recommendations are used to provide guidance to infant-food manufacturers on the composition of artificial formulas for infants that will be suitable as the sole source of nutrition. Finally, international recommendations can be used for political and medical purposes to assess the needs of infants at risk of malnutrition.

The FAO/WHO/UNU (1985) report on energy and protein requirements defines energy requirement as 'the level of energy intake from food that will balance energy expenditure when the individual has a body size and composition, and level of physical activity, consistent with long-term health; and that will allow for the maintenance of economically necessary and socially desirable physical activity'. A caveat is added for children that 'the energy requirement should include the energy needs associated with the deposition of tissues (i.e. growth) at rates consistent with good health'.

The actual FAO/WHO/UNU (1985) recommendations for food energy intake during infancy have changed substantially since the first committee report in 1950. At that time a 'blanket' figure of 800 kcal (3.35 MJ) per day during the first year of life was recommended. Subsequent reports (FAO, 1957, 1973; FAO/WHO/UNU, 1985) have refined the recommendations by giving values at more discrete age points. These recommendations are shown in Fig. 5.12. The most recent FAO/WHO/UNU recommendations are primarily based upon the data reviewed by

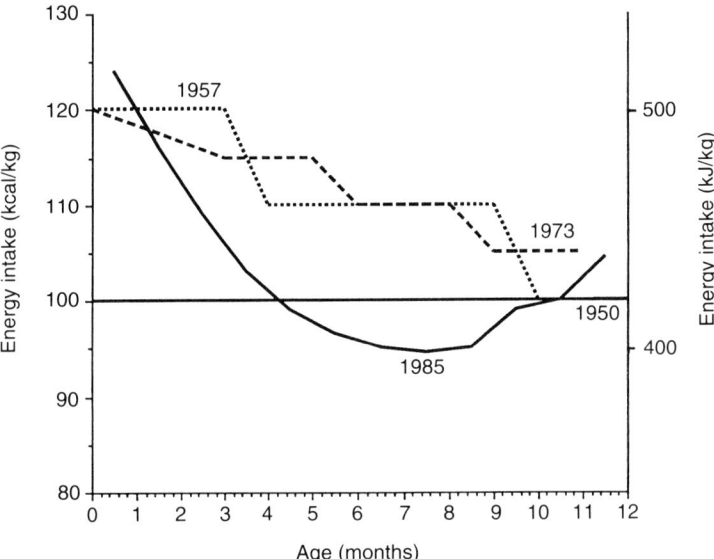

Figure 5.12 Recommendations for energy intake in the first year of life as given by various expert committees.

Whitehead *et al.* (1981). In this paper over 9000 individual measurements of food energy intake in infants were reviewed. All the studies selected for the review were carried out in Canada, Sweden, USA or the UK. No surveys from the developing countries were included, to avoid the potential complication of poor socioeconomic status.

The line of best fit through the data points should be a characteristic 'U' shape, and a quadratic equation was derived to represent the data points. The biological significance of this curve (shown in Fig. 5.12) was that energy intake was high in very early infancy owing to the high proportion of energy intake required for growth, but as this proportion diminished rapidly (see Table 5.1) energy intake decreased to reach a nadir at about 6 months of age. After this time, levels of physical activity increased, thus raising the energy requirement and hence intake of the child.

Nevertheless, the recent estimated average requirements for British infants (Department of Health, 1991) do not show the same pattern. Although requirements show a fall from 480 kJ (115 kcal)/kg per day in the first month of life, the new values do not fall as low as the FAO/WHO/UNU values, but remain constant at 397 kJ (95 kcal)/kg per day from 6 months through to 36 months of age. These data are shown in Table 5.3.

Table 5.3 The estimated average requirement of energy for children aged 0–12 months

Age (months)	Intake (kJ/kg body weight)
1	481
3	418
6	397
9	397
12	397

From Department of Health (1991).

However, all recommendations since the original 1950 FAO publication have been based upon measurements of energy *intake*, despite repeated statements by the FAO/WHO/UNU committees that recommendation should be based upon measures of *expenditure*. The problem has been, as alluded to earlier, measuring energy expenditure non-invasively in infants. The many problems inherent in assessing energy expenditure in infancy have now been overcome to a large extent, and there is a burgeoning interest in this field (Butte *et al.* 1989; Davies *et al.* 1989) using stable isotopes.

The doubly labelled water method was originally developed in the 1950s for use in small mammals and was later applied to man (Schoeller and van Santen, 1982; Coward *et al.* 1984; Klein *et al.* 1984). The principle of the method is that two stable isotopes of water ($H_2{}^{18}O$ and ^2H_2O) are administered simultaneously, and their initial enrichment and subsequent disappearance rates in a body fluid (e.g. urine or saliva) are monitored by isotope ratio mass spectrometry. The initial increase in enrichment of either isotope reflects body-water pool size (from the principle of dilution) and permits an estimation of body composition.

Subsequently, the disappearance rate of ^2H_2O reflects water output (and hence water intake); that of $^2H_2{}^{18}O$ reflects water output plus CO_2 production, because ^{18}O is free to interchange between water and CO_2 through the action of carbonic anhydrase (see Fig. 5.13). The difference between the two disappearance rates is therefore a measure of CO_2 production rate. With additional knowledge of the subject's respiratory quotient, oxygen consumption and hence energy expenditure can be calculated using a standard equation.

The doubly labelled water technique has now been used successfully in a number of studies involving infants. The common finding in all such studies is that energy expenditure values in infants are seemingly very low. Under the provocative title 'Are current dietary guidelines for young children a prescription for overfeeding?', Prentice and colleagues (1988) collated the available data at that time relating to energy expenditure

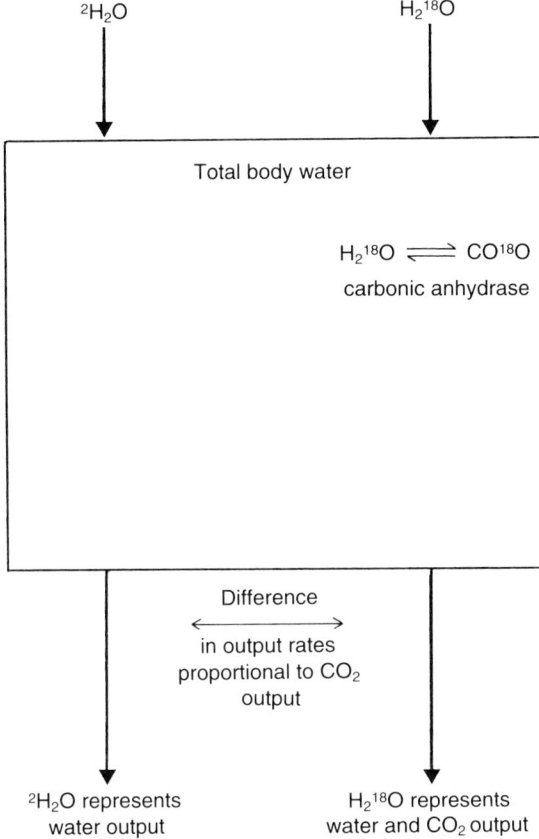

Figure 5.13 The principle of the doubly labelled water technique for measuring CO_2 production rate.

Table 5.4 The calculated energy intakes derived from measurements of energy expenditure by doubly labelled water and the difference between these and the FAO/WHO/UNU (1985) recommendations

Age (months)	'Calculated' intake (kJ/kg)	Difference from 1985 recommendations (kJ/kg)
1	460	−42
3	397	−46
6	356	−46
9	347	−59
12	347	−96

measurements carried out using stable isotopes. When energy expenditure measurements were increased to allow for energy deposited during growth, the resulting values were still markedly below the FAO/WHO/UNU (1985) recommendations. These calculated values for intake and the difference between them and the 1985 recommendations are shown in Table 5.4. The new estimates of energy requirements based on measurements using the doubly labelled water technique are closer to the observed intakes of breast-fed infants, as shown in Fig. 5.14. The FAO/WHO/UNU (1985) recommendations fall midway between intakes of infants receiving old-style full cream milk formulas, and those fed on

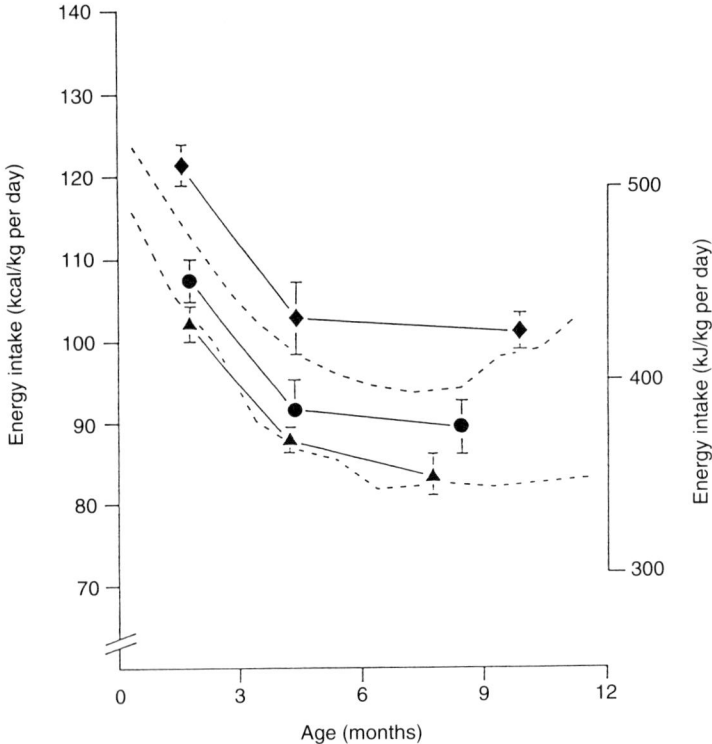

Figure 5.14 Subdivision of energy intake data according to mode of feeding, which was used as the basis of the FAO/WHO/UNU (1985) report. The upper dotted line represents the FAO/WHO/UNU (1985) recommendations and the lower dotted line new estimates of requirements derived from measurements of energy intake using the doubly labelled water technique (Prentice *et al.* 1988). Intake data are from Whitehead *et al.* (1981): ◆ old-style formulas before 1975; ● newer modified formulas; ▲ breast-fed. Values are means ± SEM.

the newer modified milk formulas. In a similar manner to the philosophy behind whether to base growth standards on the slower growth of breast-fed infants, the Department of Health's panel on dietary reference values considered that it is not necessarily appropriate to base estimates for all children on data derived from breast-fed infants. The estimated average requirements (Department of Health, 1991) are therefore for formula-fed infants *only*. They are based on the FAO/WHO/UNU (1985) values without the 5% increment that had been added to take account of a perceived underestimation of breast milk intake, and they are in line with infants fed modern formulas as shown in Fig. 5.14. It could be argued that the requirements of breast-fed infants represent the optimum as a result of natural selection in the evolution of the human race. However, breast milk production is a balance between the needs of the mother as well as the infant, and could have been limiting, in order to protect the mother, at times of food shortages. Only when further studies provide more data on the consequences of higher energy intakes in bottle-fed infants, both during infancy and in later life, will the choice of a model between breast-fed or bottle-fed infants become more sound.

As more data pertaining to energy expenditure during infancy are collected, expert committees may at last be able to reassess requirements and recommendations on that basis.

REFERENCES

Aitken, F.C. and Hytten, F.E. (1960) Infant feeding: comparison of breast and artificial feeding. *Nutrition Abstracts and Reviews*, **30**, 341–371.

Birkbeck, J.A., Buckfield, P.M. and Silva, P.A. (1985) Lack of long-term effect of the method of infant feeding on growth. *Human Nutrition: Clinical Nutrition*, **39C**, 39–44.

Butte, N.F., Wong, W., Garza, C. and Klein, P. (1989) Energy expenditure and growth of breast fed and formula fed infants (Abstract). *FASEB Journal*, **3**, A934.

Butte, N.F., Smith, O.E. and Garza, C. (1990) Energy utilization of human milk fed and formula fed infants. *American Journal of Clinical Nutrition*, **51**, 350–358.

Chandra, R. K. (1982) Physical growth of exclusively breastfed infants. *Nutrition Research*, **2**, 275–276.

Chinn, S. and Rona, R.J. (1984) The secular trend in height of primary school children in England and Scotland from 1972–1980. *Annals of Human Biology*, **11**, 1–16.

Cole, T.J. (1988) Fitting smooth centile curves to reference data. *Journal of the Royal Statistical Society, Series A*, **151**, 385–418.

Coward, W.A., Prentice, A.M., Murgatroyd, P.R. *et al.* (1984) Measurement of CO_2 production rates in man using $^2H_2{}^{18}O$ labelled H_2O): comparison between calorimeter and isotope values. In *Human Energy Metabolism: Physical Activity and Energy Expenditure Measurements in Epidemiological Research Based upon*

Direct and Indirect Calorimetry (European Nutrition Report no. 5), pp. 126–128 (ed A.J.H. van Es). Den Haag: CIP-gegeres koninklijke.

Czajka-Narins, D.M. and Jung, E. (1986) Physical growth of breast-fed and formula-fed infants from birth to age two years. *Nutrition Research*, 6, 753–762.

Davies, D.P. (1973) Plasma osmolality and feeding practices of healthy infants in the first three months of life. *British Medical Journal*, 2, 340–342.

Davies, P.S.W. (1991) The measurement of physical activity in children using the doubly labelled water technique. In *Physical Activity and Health*, pp. 45–56 (ed. N. Norgan). Cambridge: Cambridge University Press.

Davies, P.S.W., Ewing, G. and Lucas, A. (1989) Energy expenditure in early infancy. *British Journal of Nutrition*, 62, 621–629.

Department of Health (UK) (1991) *Dietary Reference Values for Food Energy and Nutrients for the United Kingdom*. Reports on Health and Social Subjects no. 41. London: HMSO.

Dewey, K.G., Heinig, M.J., Nommsen, L.A. and Lonnerdal, B. (1990) Low energy intakes and growth velocities of breast-fed infants: are there functional consequences? In *Activity, Energy Expenditure and Energy Requirements of Infants and Children. Proceedings of an IDECG Workshop*, pp. 35–44 (eds B. Schurch and N.S. Scrimshaw). Lausanne: IDECG/Nestlé Foundation.

DHSS (UK) (1974) *Present Day Practice in Infant Feeding*. Reports on Health and Social Subjects no. 9. London: HMSO.

DHSS (UK) (1988) *Present Day Practice in Infant Feeding: Third Report*. Reports on Health and Social Subjects no. 32. London: HMSO.

Emery, J.L., Waite, A.J., Carpenter, R.G. *et al.* (1985) Apnoea monitors compared with weighing scales for siblings after cot death. *Archives of Diseases in Childhood*, 60, 1055–1060.

FAO (1950) *Calorie Requirements: Report of the Committee on Calorie Requirements*. FAO Nutritional Studies no. 5. Rome: Food and Agricultural Organization.

FAO (1957) *Calorie Requirements: Report of the Second Committee on Calorie Requirements*. FAO Nutritional Studies no. 15. Rome: Food and Agricultural Organization.

FAO (1973) *Energy and Protein Requirements*. FAO Nutrition Meeting Report Series no. 52; WHO Technical Report Series no. 522. Rome: Food and Agricultural Organization; Geneva: World Health Organization.

FAO/WHO/UNU (1985) *Energy and Protein Requirements*. WHO Technical Report Series no. 724. Geneva: World Health Organization.

Fomon, S.J., Haschke, F., Ziegler, E.E. and Nelson, S.E. (1982) Body composition of reference children from birth to age 10 years. *American Journal of Clinical Nutrition*, 35, 1169–1175.

Gracey, M. (1987) Normal growth and nutrition. *World Review of Nutrition and Dietetics*, 49, 160–210.

Hamill, P.V.V., Drizd, T.A., Johnson, C.L. *et al.* (1977) *NCHS Growth Curves for Children, Birth to 18 Years*. US Department of Health, Education and Welfare Publications No. PHD 78–1650. Hyattsville, MD: National Center for Health Statistics.

Hamosh, M. (1988) Does infant nutrition affect adiposity and cholesterol levels in the adult? *Journal of Pediatric Gastroenterology and Nutrition*, 7, 10–16.

Hitchcock, N.E., Gracey, M. and Gilmour, A. (1985) The growth of breastfed and artificially fed infants from birth to twelve months. *Acta Paediatrica Scandinavica*, 74, 240–245.

Hutchinson-Smith, B. (1973) Skinfold thickness in infancy in relation to birth-weight. *Developmental Medicine: Childhood Neurology*, **15**, 628–634.

Klein, P.D., James, W.P.T., Wong, W.W. *et al.* (1984) Calorimetric validation of the doubly labelled water method for the determination of energy expenditure in man. *Human Nutrition: Clinical Nutrition*, **38C**, 95–106.

Kramer, M.S., Barr, R.G., Leduc, D.G., Boisjoly, C., McVey-White, L. and Pless, I.B. (1985) Determinants of weight and adiposity in the first year of life. *Journal of Pediatrics*, **106**, 10–14.

Martin, J. and White, A. (1988) *Infant Feeding 1985*. London: HMSO.

Ministry of Health (UK) (1959) *Standards of Normal Weight in Infancy*. Reports on Health and Social Subjects no. 99. London: HMSO.

Paul, A.A., Whitehead, R.G. and Black, A.E. (1990) Energy intake and growth from two months to three years in children initially breastfed. *Journal of Human Nutrition and Dietetics*, **3**, 117–130.

Pomerance, H.H. (1987) Growth in breast-fed children. *Human Biology*, **59**, 687–693.

Poskitt, E.M.E. and Cole, T.J. (1977) Do fat babies stay fat? *Lancet*, **i**, 7–9.

Prentice, A., Lucas, A., Vasquez-Velasquez, L. *et al.* (1988) Are current dietary guidelines for young children a prescription for overfeeding? *Lancet*, **ii**, 1066–1068.

Roche, A.F., Guo, S. and Moore, W.M. (1989) Weight and recumbent length from 1 to 12 mo of age: reference data for 1-mo increments. *American Journal of Clinical Nutrition*, **49**, 599–607.

Roede, M.J. and van Wieringen, J.C. (1985) Growth diagrams 1980. Netherlands third nationwide survey. *Tijdschrifst v Societie Gezondheim*, **63**, 1–34.

Salmenpera, L., Perheentupa, J. and Siimes, M.A. (1985) Exclusively breastfed healthy infants grow slower than reference values. *Pediatric Research*, **19**, 307–312.

Schoeller, D.A. and van Santen, E. (1982) Measurement of energy expenditure in humans by doubly labelled water. *Journal of Applied Physiology*, **53**, 955–959.

Schofield, W.N., Schofield, C. and James, W.P.T. (1985) Basal metabolic rate: review and prediction, together with an annotated bibliography of source material. *Human Nutrition: Clinical Nutrition*, **39C** (Suppl. 1), 5–41.

Schluter, J., Funfack, W., Pachaly, J. and Weber, B. (1976) Development of subcutaneous fat in infancy. Standards for tricipital, subscapular and suprailiacal skinfolds in German infants. *European Journal of Pediatrics*, **123**, 255–267.

Sullivan, K., Trowbridge, F., Gorstein, J. and Pradilla, A. (1991) Growth references. *Lancet*, **337**, 1420–1421.

Taitz, L.S. (1971) Infantile overnutrition among artificially fed infants in the Sheffield region. *British Medical Journal*, **i**, 315–316.

Tanner, J.M. and Whitehouse, R.M. (1962) Standards for subcutaneous fat in British children. *British Medical Journal*, **i**, 446–450.

Tanner, J.M. and Whitehouse, R.H. (1975) Revised standards for triceps and subscapular skinfolds in British children. *Archives of Diseases in Childhood*, **50**, 142–145.

Tanner, J.M., Whitehouse, R.H. and Takaishi, M. (1966) Standards from birth to maturity for height, weight, height velocity and weight velocity: British children 1965. *Archives of Diseases in Childhood*, **41**, 613–635.

Waterlow, J.C. (1988) Basic concepts in the determination of nutritional requirements of normal infants. In *Nutrition During Infancy*, pp. 1–20 (eds R.C. Tsang and B.L. Nicols). Philadelphia, PA: Hanley & Belfus.

Waterlow, J.C., Ashworth, A. and Griffiths, M. (1980) Faltering in infant growth in less developed countries. *Lancet*, **ii**, 1176–1178.

Whitehead, R.G. and Paul, A.A. (1984) Growth charts and the assessment of infant feeding practices in the western world and in developing countries. *Early Human Development*, **9**, 187–207.

Whitehead, R.G. and Paul, A.A. (1987) Changes in infant feeding in Britain during the last century. In *Infant Nutrition and Cardiovascular Disease* (Scientific Report no. 8), pp. 1–10. Southampton: MRC Environmental Epidemiology Unit.

Whitehead, R.G., Paul, A.A. and Cole, T.J. (1981) A critical analysis of measured food energy intakes during infancy and early childhood in comparison with current international recommendations. *Journal of Human Nutrition*, **35**, 339–348

Whitehead, R.G., Paul, A. A. and Ahmed, E.A. (1988) United Kingdom Department of Health and Social Security 'Present Day Infant Feeding Practice' and its influence on infant growth. In *The Physiology of Human Growth* (Proceedings of the Society for the Study of Human Biology no. 29), pp. 69–79 (eds J.M. Tanner and M.A. Preece). Cambridge: Cambridge University Press.

Whitehead, R.G., Paul, A.A. and Cole, T.J. (1989) Diet and the growth of healthy infants. *Journal of Human Nutrition and Dietetics*, **2**, 73–84.

WHO (1978) *A Growth Chart for International Use in Maternal and Child Welfare*. Geneva: World Health Organization.

Yeung, D.L. (1983) *Infant Nutrition: A Study of Feeding Practices and Growth from Birth to 18 Months*. Ontario: Canadian Public Health Association.

6
Infant feeding and infectious disease

Suzanne Filteau and Andrew Tomkins
Centre for International Child Health, Institute of Child Health, London, UK

INTRODUCTION

Infectious diseases take the lives of many infants and young children in developing countries. Furthermore, the adverse effects of infection linger even among the survivors who may suffer growth faltering and its associated risks, including, in the short term, increased susceptibility to infection (Tomkins and Watson, 1989) and, in the long term, decreased life-long productivity (Gopalan, 1988). Because of the devastating effects of infectious disease, much research has dealt with possible means of prevention of infection, including immunization and improved sanitation, water supplies and personal hygiene. One factor which appears to have an important influence on an infant's risk of and response to an infection is the infant's diet. Infant feeding practices and their relation to infectious disease are the subject of this review, with particular emphasis on the role of breast feeding but also with some discussion of weaning foods.

EPIDEMIOLOGICAL ASSOCIATION BETWEEN BREAST FEEDING AND REDUCED INFECTION

A large number of studies investigating infectious disease morbidity and mortality in developing countries have convincingly demonstrated a protective effect of breast feeding. Several reviews have summarized this copious literature (Jason *et al.* 1984; JHU/WHO, 1989). In spite of

Infant Nutrition. Edited by A.F. Walker and B.A. Rolls.
Published in 1994 by Chapman & Hall, London.
ISBN 0 412 59140 5.

problems with methods in some of the earlier studies (Jason *et al.* 1984), the evidence justifies active promotion of breast feeding in developing countries, based on concerns of infectious disease alone, irrespective of socioeconomic or other factors which further strengthen this recommendation.

However, these studies in developing countries give little information as to how breast feeding protects against infectious disease. Two types of mechanisms can be postulated: a direct protection due to intrinsic factors in breast milk, or an indirect effect due mainly to the fact that breast feeding delays and reduces the infant's exposure to potentially contaminated weaning foods (Clemens *et al.* 1993). Information concerning the relative importance of these direct and indirect effects can be gleaned by comparing studies of breast feeding and infection from industrialized and less developed countries or by investigating infectious disease in partly breast-fed infants in various environments, as will be discussed below.

Evidence from industrialized countries for an infection-preventing effect of breast feeding is much less definitive than that from developing countries (Bauchner *et al.* 1986). This ambiguity may result from the difficulty of conducting adequately controlled tests of a hypothesis for which experimental randomization is unethical and for which any difference between groups is likely to be small. In addition, it is possible that protective effects occur only over a narrow age range or only for particular pathogens and such effects would be hard to discern in small studies or in those where all ages or all infections were considered together. Nevertheless, recent studies that incorporated recommended design features (Bauchner *et al.* 1986) support a small but real protective effect of breast feeding even in clean environments in industrialized countries. For example, breast feeding reduced the incidence of gastrointestinal illness in infants in Scotland (Howie *et al.* 1990), and of lower respiratory tract infection in infants in the USA (Wright *et al.* 1989). Breast feeding had no effect on the incidence of rotavirus infection in American infants but decreased the duration and severity of the disease (Duffy *et al.* 1986). The mechanism of this effect is unknown and may not necessarily be related to improved immune functions in breast-fed infants. Improved nutrition or a direct beneficial effect of food on the gut may play a role since it has been shown that the intake of breast milk decreases less than the intake of other foods during acute diarrhoea in infants (Brown *et al.* 1990). In general, these studies suggest an intrinsic protective effect of breast milk since alternative or complementary foods in industrialized countries are not normally grossly contaminated. Furthermore, these results support promotion of breast feeding in industrialized as well as in developing countries.

In addition to the intrinsic protective effect of breast milk seen in industrialized countries, the much greater protective effect of breast feeding in developing countries presumably results from an additive or synergistic combination with extrinsic factors. That is, it is likely that much of the protection from infectious disease by breast feeding in developing countries is due to the reduction and postponement of the consumption of unhygienic weaning foods until the infant's own defences have had a chance to mature. An additional interpretation is that the innate protective effects of breast milk are more easily demonstrated against a backdrop of high risk of infection. Risk factors for infection include living in poverty in developing countries, prematurity and low birth weight. For example, in the study of lower respiratory tract infection in the USA (Wright *et al.* 1989), breast feeding had the greatest protective effect in infants who were Mexican-American and who shared a room – factors suggestive of lower socioeconomic status and crowding. Several studies involving high-risk premature or low birth weight infants have shown a clear protective effect of breast feeding on infection (Jason *et al.* 1984).

Another way to determine the relative importance of intrinsic and extrinsic factors in the protection against infectious disease provided by breast feeding is to consider the partly breast-fed infant. If intrinsic factors in breast milk are more important, then the risk of infection of the partly breast-fed infant should approach that of the exclusively breast-fed infant. If, on the other hand, breast feeding protects mainly by reducing exposure to contaminated supplementary foods, infection rates in the partly breast-fed infant should be similar to those in the completely weaned infant. Unfortunately, not all researchers in the field have clearly distinguished between full and partial breast feeding nor have they always indicated the nature of alternative and supplementary foods and their microbiological contamination. However, some recent studies merit consideration. In developing countries the risk of infection for partly breast-fed infants is generally intermediate between the risks for exclusively breast-fed and completely weaned infants (Victora *et al.* 1987; Brown *et al.* 1989), although the risk of *Giardia* infection was similar in totally and partly breast-fed infants and less than that in artificially fed infants in Gabon (Gendrel *et al.* 1989). An association was seen between the degree of risk and the degree of supplementation with foods other than breast milk in that risks for gastrointestinal and respiratory illnesses were lower in infants who received only liquids in addition to breast milk than in those who also received other milks or solids (Brown *et al.* 1989). The increased risk of diarrhoea for both partly breast-fed and non-breast-fed infants was greater than that of respiratory or other infections, as would be expected if increased exposure to food pathogens were the major problem in these children (Victora *et al.* 1987).

An unusual controlled experimental trial of human milk or formula feeding of high-risk low birth weight infants in India provided further information concerning the partly breast-fed infant (Narayanan *et al.* 1984). Infants were randomly allocated to receive either raw or pasteurized human milk either alone or in combination with formula. Formula feeding alone was not used since previous work by this group indicated a very high incidence of infection in infants receiving formula alone, confirming that in this environment these infants were at high risk. Formula feeding increased the incidence of infection even though microbiological analysis indicated the formula was sterile. In addition, there was a synergy between pasteurization of the human milk and addition of formula, since either treatment alone induced a relatively small increase in infection rates compared with feeding with raw milk only, but a large increase was seen when both treatments were combined. Perhaps the amount of human milk given to the infants receiving mixed feed did not reach some necessary threshold, particularly when the concentrations of some intrinsic protective factors were decreased by pasteurization.

In industrialized countries, however, partial breast feeding appears to carry little risk compared with total breast feeding. In Scotland no significant difference in risk of gastrointestinal illness was seen between infants either fully or partly breast-fed for the first 13 weeks of life (Howie *et al.* 1990). In the study showing no effect of breast feeding on the incidence of rotavirus infection in American infants, the decrease in severity of the disease was similar in totally and partly breast-fed infants (Duffy *et al.* 1986). These results suggest that in a clean environment where supplementary foods are not microbially contaminated, their addition to the infant's diet has little effect on infectious disease incidence and that there exists a threshold of breast milk intake beyond which there is no further protective effect.

Breast feeding and maternal infection, including AIDS

The above information has implied that breast milk, unlike alternative foods, is not itself a source of infection. However, what about the case where the mother is infected? In the study of Narayanan and co-workers (1984) a major reason for artificially feeding the infants was maternal infection. Potentially pathogenic organisms could be cultured from 15% of the breast milk samples from these women. In spite of this contamination, breast milk was more protective against infection than sterile formula and was more effective raw than pasteurized. Presumably the intrinsic protective factors in breast milk are potent enough to overcome at least modest microbial contamination of the milk.

One maternal infection for which the arguments for and against breast

feeding have recently been debated is human immunodeficiency virus (HIV) infection. Many are concerned about possible transmission of HIV by an infected mother to her own infant or by banked milk from an infected donor to other infants. The risk of transmission by breast feeding is estimated to be 14% (Ziegler, 1993). This risk must be balanced in individual circumstances with the risks associated with bottle feeding. In areas where there is a high risk of other infections which could aggravate the condition of an infant already potentially infected with HIV *in utero*, and where safe, affordable alternative foods are unavailable, breast feeding will remain the safest option. In industrialized countries where formula is safer and more readily available, the potential risks of both bottle and breast feeding should be explained as clearly as possible to an HIV-infected mother. Finally, in the event of maternal HIV infection or other problems with breast feeding, it would be useful to have a safe supply of banked milk. A combination of pasteurization to destroy the virus (Editorial, 1988) and screening and HIV testing of donors should make the risk of HIV infection from banked milk negligible.

Duration of breast feeding and protection from infection

Whereas few would deny that breast feeding should be encouraged for all newborn infants, there remains some debate as to the optimum time breast feeding should be continued. In industrialized countries, where safe, clean, nutritionally adequate supplementary or alternative foods are readily available, no improved disease resistance was conferred by breast feeding beyond 13 weeks (Howie *et al.* 1990) or 4 months (Wright *et al.* 1989). Furthermore, breast feeding for 13 weeks protected the infant even after complete weaning (Howie *et al.* 1990). It is likely that by this time the breast-fed infant's gut and immune system have matured to the point that they provide a considerable defence. Similar careful studies are needed to determine whether such a threshold exists in other environments as well.

In developing countries where good clean alternatives to breast milk are less readily available, the question of when to supplement or wean the infant is considerably more complex and has been dubbed the 'weaning dilemma' (Underwood, 1985). Postponement of the introduction of contaminated alternative foods seems reasonable, but it is important to mention that prolonged breast feeding, continuing into the second year of life, has been associated with poor nutritional status of the infant, even when other foods were also given (Victora *et al.* 1984; Brakohiapa *et al.* 1988). Poverty may be a confounding factor; that is, the long-term breast-fed infants are often from the poorest families (Victora *et al.* 1984) and may be the most susceptible to other causes of growth faltering including

infection due to poor hygiene or crowding, lack of medical care and neglect as well as having little access to clean nutritious weaning foods. Alternatively, malnutrition in these children may result from low food intake (Brakohiapa *et al.* 1988) due to poor appetite for complementary weaning foods which may be monotonous or bland (Underwood, 1985). Infants may need to be acquainted with a variety of tastes and food textures in order to stimulate appetite for weaning foods before they become nutritionally essential (Underwood, 1985). Thus a dilemma arises. Whereas early in life high-risk infants appear to benefit most from the protective effects of breast feeding, such benefit either does not continue into the second year of life or is overwhelmed by other factors. However, those high-risk infants are likely to suffer at weaning owing to unavailability of clean, nutritionally adequate weaning foods. More research needs to be conducted concerning breast feeding and risk of infection in older infants and the health consequences of different weaning practices need to be more clearly evaluated. Attention needs to be directed towards development and provision of appropriate, locally available, low-cost weaning foods.

BREAST MILK AND ENHANCEMENT OF IMMUNITY IN INFANTS

The epidemiological associations between breast feeding and decreased morbidity and mortality from infectious disease have stimulated much fruitful research into immunological mechanisms for these associations. Most research has concentrated on passive immunity provided to the infant by immunological factors found in breast milk. Such passive immunity has been considered as a continuation after birth of that provided prenatally by immunoglobulin G (IgG) transfer across the placenta. The subject has been recently reviewed (Akre, 1989). Tables 6.1 and 6.2 list the various soluble and cellular components of breast milk that are believed to contribute to protection of infants from infectious disease. Although quantities of most factors are much greater in colostrum than in mature milk, the volume of the latter is so much greater that the infant's intake varies relatively little for the first few weeks.

Secretory IgA (sIgA), which consists of a dimer of IgA plus a protein of epithelial origin known as secretory component, is often considered the most important immunological factor in milk and has been the subject of the most extensive research in the field. The quantities in milk represent a large immunoglobulin dose for the infant (Akre, 1989). A large proportion of the infant's IgA intake appears intact in the faeces (Prentice *et al.* 1987), illustrating (1) the resistance of sIgA to degradation within the gut lumen, (2) the unavailability of some sIgA (which comprises about

Table 6.1 Soluble anti-infective factors in human milk

Factor	Concentration		Postulated function	References
	Colostrum	Mature milk		
sIgA (μg/ml)	2000	400–1000	Prevention of attachment of pathogens and toxins to intestinal wall	Cruz et al. (1982); Goldman et al. (1982); Prentice et al. (1983)
Lactoferrin (μg/ml)	5000	500–2500	Withholding iron from micro-organisms	Goldman et al. (1982); Prentice et al. (1983); Hennart et al. (1991)
Lysozyme (μg/ml)	100–150	50–300	Disruption of bacterial cell walls	Andersson et al. (1985). Viverge et al. (1985) Coppa (1990)
Oligosacch-arides (μg/ml)	10	5–8	Prevention of bacterial adhesion; promotion of bifidobacteria	Petschow and Talbott (1991)
Nucleotides (μg/ml)	–	70–200	Enhancement of immune system development; promotion of bifido-bacteria	Carver et al. (1991) Quan et al. (1990

Table 6.2 Immune cells in human milk

Cell type	No. per ml		Postulated function	References
	Colostrum	Mature milk		
Macro-phages	10^6	10^4	Release of synthesized or previously ingested antibodies and regulatory molecules	Crago et al. (1979); Goldman et al. (1982); Blau et al. (1983)
Neutro-phils	10^6	10^4	Phagocytosis + microbicide?	Crago et al. (1979); Goldman et al. (1982)
Lympho-cytes	10^5–10^6	10^3–10^4	Antibody production? Transfer of immunological memory? Stimulation of immune system development?	Ogra and Ogra (1978); Goldman et al. (1982); Bertotto et al. (1990)

10% of the total protein in milk) as a protein source for the infant (Hambraeus *et al.* 1984), and (3) the existence of a major function for sIgA within the gut. Secretory IgA is believed to protect the infant mainly by preventing adherence of pathogens to the intestinal wall, an early step in infection (Editorial, 1981). Similarly, sIgA may prevent toxins from binding to the gut wall (Stoliar *et al.* 1976). Antibody responses, like other lymphocyte responses, can be augmented by vaccination or prior infection with a particular infectious agent. Such specific sIgA antibodies to various pathogens to which the mother has been exposed are found in milk, thus protecting the infant against relevant environmental pathogens (Stoliar *et al.* 1976; Davis *et al.* 1982).

Lactoferrin is a specific high-affinity iron-binding protein comprising about 20% of the total protein in human milk (Prentice *et al.* 1983, 1987; Goldman *et al.* 1982). It competes effectively with intestinal microbes for any available iron and thus helps limit microbial growth (Weinberg, 1984). As with sIgA, intact lactoferrin can be found in the stools of breast-fed infants (Prentice *et al.* 1987), indicating that it at least partly escapes digestion and that its function within the gut lumen is important.

Lysozyme is an enzyme found in secreted fluids such as sweat, saliva and tears (Roitt *et al.* 1989). It can damage bacterial cell walls and thus is bacteriostatic. Its concentration in milk increases steadily as lactation progresses even into the second year (Prentice *et al.* 1983; Goldman *et al.* 1982; Hennart *et al.* 1991).

In addition to these well established antimicrobial factors in milk, there exist less well defined soluble milk components which also appear to protect infants from infectious disease. For example, *Giardia lamblia* was killed by exposure to human milk *in vitro*, possibly through the action of bile salt-stimulated lipase, an enzyme found in human but not cows' milk (Gillin *et al.* 1983). Milk fractions that have been depleted of antibodies can still block adhesion of bacteria to epithelial cells (Andersson *et al.* 1985; Coppa *et al.* 1990). This activity has been attributed to oligo-saccharides (sugars) which could competitively inhibit binding of bacteria to epithelial glycolipids. The oligosaccharide profile of the urine of breast-fed infants corresponds to that in their mother's milk (Coppa *et al.* 1990). Thus it is possible that not only the epithelium of the intestine but also that of the urinary tract is protected by milk from colonization by bacteria (Coppa *et al.* 1990).

In addition to these soluble antimicrobial factors, breast milk contains leucocytes which may also contribute to protection of the infant from infection. The number of leucocytes per millilitre varies widely, not only among individuals but also within an individual on consecutive days (Crago *et al.* 1979).

Macrophages are a type of phagocytic leucocyte: that is, they ingest invading pathogens and subject them to an assortment of toxic chemicals, particularly active oxygen metabolites (Roitt *et al.* 1989). Systemic macrophages secrete a wide range of products, both antimicrobial ones such as components of the complement system, and regulatory ones such as interleukin 1 which functions as a hormone in the immune and other physiological systems (Roitt *et al.* 1989). Although macrophages are usually thought to protect mainly internal organs rather than mucosal surfaces, they are also one of the predominant milk leucocytes (Crago *et al.* 1979; Blau *et al.* 1983). Milk macrophages differ in some respects from macrophages derived from blood monocytes (Crago *et al.* 1979). For example, many are engorged with lipid and appear to have ingested various milk proteins since they contain proteins such as sIgA and lactalbumin which are not normally found in systemic macrophages (Crago *et al.* 1979). In spite of these differences, milk macrophages *in vitro* were capable of carrying out similar functions and synthesizing similar products to blood-derived macrophages (Blau *et al.* 1983). They are likely to be the milk leucocytes that secrete interleukin 1 *in vitro* (Munoz *et al.* 1990). However, since most milk macrophages could not survive pH 3.5 (Blau *et al.* 1983), their ability to function after passage through the stomach is questionable. They may still be able to release immunologically active factors either synthesized or previously ingested by them.

Neutrophils are also numerous in colostrum and milk (Crago *et al.* 1979; Goldman *et al.* 1982) but appear to have been relatively little studied. In adults these phagocytic cells provide the main cellular defence of the skin and mucosal surfaces and are the first cells to appear when these physical barriers are broken. Like milk macrophages, milk neutrophils contain large lipid-filled vacuoles (Crago *et al.* 1979). Unlike either milk macrophages or blood neutrophils which are highly motile cells, milk neutrophils do not appear to migrate either spontaneously or in response to chemotactic agents (Ozkaragoz *et al.* 1988). Much remains to be learned about the functions of these cells.

Lymphocytes comprise 5–10% of the milk leucocyte population (Crago *et al.* 1979; Goldman *et al.* 1986). About half the lymphocytes are T-cells, that is, thymus-dependent lymphocytes that carry out cell-mediated immune functions and also regulate many other aspects of immunity including antibody production. Another third are B-cells, the lymphocytes that synthesize antibody, and the remainder are null (non-T, non-B) cells (Diaz-Jouanen and Williams, 1974; Saha *et al.* 1987). Unlike blood B-cells, which have mainly surface IgG, a large proportion of milk B-cells bear surface IgA, reflecting the predominance of IgA at mucosal surfaces and in secreted fluids (Diaz-Jouanen and Williams, 1974). Whether these B-cells continue to secrete IgA after ingestion by the infant is debatable

since most of the IgA in faeces of breast-fed infants (Prentice *et al.* 1987) or secreted *in vitro* by colostral cells (Goldblum *et al.* 1975) is secretory IgA whereas lymphocytes themselves cannot make secretory component. It appears more likely that the IgA provided to the infant is either free in solution or else inside the milk macrophages (Crago *et al.* 1979). Thus the function of the milk B-cells remains unclear.

Many authors have noted that, relative to blood T-cells, milk T-cells respond only weakly to polyclonal mitogens (Diaz-Jouanen and Williams 1974; Ogra and Ogra, 1978). Such proliferative responses are often suggested to reflect immunological capability, even though most researchers realize this interpretation is a gross oversimplification. A possible explanation for the low responses of milk T-cells is that these cells appear to be memory T-cells that have been previously exposed to an antigen and respond to mitogens less well than do immunologically naive T-cells (Bertotto *et al.* 1990). Presumably the milk T-cells function to protect the infant from pathogens to which the mother has been exposed or to transmit immunological memory to the infant, rather than to respond to new antigens. Transfer through breast milk of responsiveness to tuberculin has been documented (Schlesinger and Covelli, 1977). The mechanism of such memory transfer is unknown but may involve cytokines, that is, hormones secreted by T-cells or other leucocytes. For example, milk T-cells can produce interferon in quantities at least as great as can blood lymphocytes (Keller *et al.* 1981).

This postulated effect of milk leucocyte cytokines on the infant's immune system represents a more active role of breast milk factors in the infant's immunological development and resistance to infection than has often been considered. Most investigators have emphasized passive protection of the infant, for example by sIgA preventing adherence of bacteria to the gut. However, newer research suggests that breast feeding may enhance development of the infant's immune system, for example, by promotion of early antibody production.

Urinary concentrations of sIgA were higher in infants fed on human milk rather than formula (Prentice, 1987; Goldblum *et al.* 1989). Secretory IgA was measured in urine rather than faeces, saliva or nasal washings since urine is produced at a site remote from the immune factors in the milk or formula itself. Additional evidence that the urinary sIgA was produced by the infants themselves is that urinary concentrations did not correlate with dietary intake and that sIgA is too large to be normally filtered by the kidneys (Prentice, 1987; Goldblum *et al.* 1989). The increased antibody production by some breast-fed infants may be due to soluble factors in human milk (Pittard and Bill, 1979; Juto, 1985). Interleukin 1 in milk is relatively acid-resistant and may survive passage through the infant's stomach and promote immune functions

(Munoz *et al.* 1990). Not all researchers have found greater levels of serum or secreted antibodies in breast-fed than bottle-fed infants (Stephens *et al.* 1984; Ostergaard, 1985). Presumably some of the variation in results is due to varying antigen exposure of the infants, which would tend to increase immunoglobulin synthesis (Stephens *et al.* 1984).

As regards development of other aspects of immunity than antibody synthesis, lymphocyte subpopulation percentages of 6-month-old breast-fed infants resembled adult percentages somewhat more closely than did percentages in formula-fed infants (Carver *et al.* 1991). *In vitro* proliferation of blood lymphocytes was higher in breast-fed infants of less than 6 weeks of age but higher in formula-fed infants at 3–9 months of age (Juto *et al.* 1982; Stephens *et al.* 1986). It is likely that here also there is a balance of effects between immune factors in breast milk and the higher antigen exposure of formula-fed infants. Finally, a recent report suggests that nucleotides may be factors in breast milk that increase some infant immune functions, for example, blood lymphocyte interleukin 2 production and natural killer cell activity (Carver *et al.* 1989).

Important components of host defences generally rather neglected by immunologists are the skin and mucosal epithelia. In addition to the physical barriers provided by the skin and mucosae, the biochemical environment at these surfaces, for example, the low pH in the stomach, tends to be inimical to microbes. Breast milk may enhance resistance to infectious disease by promoting such non-specific defences. Milk contains a number of hormones and growth factors that contribute to the protection of the infant by promoting development of the gastrointestinal tract (Walker, 1985; Gaull *et al.* 1985). The intestinal epithelium as it matures becomes more able to protect itself against pathogens and recover from a pathogenic insult. With maturity, the epithelium is better able to degrade macromolecules and prevent their absorption which could lead to illness or allergic responses (Walker, 1985). The best recognized growth-promoting agent in human milk is epidermal growth factor but some other growth factors appear also to be involved (Carpenter, 1980). For example, dietary nucleotide supplements increased intestinal villus density and crypt depth in mice (Quan *et al.* 1990).

It has long been recognized that ill-defined factors in human milk influence the colonization of the infant's intestine, favouring non-pathogenic bifidobacteria (lactobacilli). These bacteria, by fermenting lactose, reduce the pH of the intestinal lumen and thus inhibit the growth of yeast and certain pathogenic Gram-negative bacteria (Akre, 1989). Factors in both the protein and non-protein nitrogen fractions, for example oligosaccharides (Petschow and Talbott, 1991) and nucleotides (Quan *et al.* 1990), appear responsible for the bifidobacteria-promoting activity of human milk.

Finally, some researchers have investigated whether the mother's nutritional status influences the levels of various protective factors in her milk. Milk volume may be less in undernourished than well nourished mothers (Jelliffe and Jelliffe, 1978). In addition, the concentrations of certain immune components, for example colostral leucocytes but not their subset percentages (Saha *et al.* 1987), sIgA (Cruz *et al.* 1982; Chang, 1990), and lysozyme (Chang, 1990), may be lower in milk from undernourished mothers. However, in general, comparable amounts of most immune factors are found in the milk of well nourished and undernourished mothers and high-energy supplements have little effect on levels of immunoglobulins, lactoferrin, lysozyme or complement components in milk (Prentice *et al.* 1983; Herias *et al.* 1993). Furthermore, in view of the wide range of normal milk concentrations of these immune factors (Crago *et al.* 1979; Cruz *et al.* 1982; Prentice *et al.* 1983), it is unclear whether the occasional decreased level of some component is of any physiological significance in terms of protection of the infant. The existence in normal milk of an excess of immune factors is supported by the evidence cited in the previous section that in developed countries partial breast feeding is as protective as total breast feeding.

WEANING FOODS AND INFECTION

The time of introduction of weaning foods will depend on many factors not directly related to the needs of the infant, including standard cultural practices, the need of the mother to return to work, and child care arrangements. However, at some point all infants will need access to nutritionally adequate, hygienic weaning foods. In industrialized countries a wide range of such products are commercially available. Introduction of these is usually recommended when the infant is 4–6 months old. Prior to this time the infant's ability to swallow solids has not developed and his gastrointestinal tract is still somewhat permeable, which may increase the risk of developing allergies (Walker, 1985). Breast feeding at least partly until this age would reach the threshold for protection against infection as discussed above.

Since weaning – the introduction of solid foods – should not normally be delayed beyond 4–6 months, appropriate weaning foods need to be determined. Two main features of these foods must be considered: nutritional adequacy and microbiological purity. Both these targets may be difficult to meet in poor families. At least for nutritional adequacy the target is relatively well defined (Walker, 1990) and it is possible in theory to develop combinations of locally available foods that meet the infant's energy, protein and micronutrient requirements. Poverty and ignorance, however, may result in nutritionally inadequate weaning foods which

could lead to malnutrition and the associated increased risk of infection.

Nutritional adequacy of infant foods

It is generally considered axiomatic that breast milk is the ideal food for infants and that infant nutritional requirements can be determined from the intake of completely breast-fed infants. Nevertheless, occasionally concern is raised about the adequacy of particular nutrients in breast milk. For example, iron in breast milk is bound to lactoferrin and thus is not very available so that breast-fed infants lose considerably more iron than they absorb (Weinberg, 1984). This iron loss appears normal, however, and iron supplementation may increase infection (Kuvibidila, 1987). Another example is that, despite widespread belief that water supplementation is required to maintain adequate hydration in infants in hot climates, breast milk alone appears sufficient (Sachdev *et al.* 1991). In fact, water supplementation of these infants may prove hazardous by decreasing breast milk intake and increasing exposure to water-borne pathogens (Sachdev *et al.* 1991).

It is less clear whether breast milk alone is adequate for premature infants (Lucas, 1986). These infants have lower stores of iron (Lucas, 1986) and vitamin A (Zachman, 1989) than full-term infants and may also be at increased risk of developing zinc deficiency (Hambidge, 1986). Supplementation of pre-term infants with these micronutrients may prove beneficial. For example, vitamin A supplements may promote repair of lung damage in premature infants (Zachman, 1989) which would help prevent invasion by respiratory pathogens.

In many developing countries a major obstacle to providing adequate nutrients and energy to infants at weaning is the high viscosity or bulk of the traditional weaning foods (Walker, 1990). These foods are generally starchy porridges with low energy densities such that unreasonably large amounts would need to be consumed by the infant to meet his energy requirements. Energy density can be improved by addition of sugar or oils to the porridge. Alternatively, techniques such as seed germination and fermentation can be used to decrease the viscosity of the porridge so that it becomes more acceptable to infants (Walker, 1990). This may be particularly important for sick infants who often have difficulty swallowing bulky foods.

The particular nutritional requirements for optimum resistance to infection in weaned infants have been studied for relatively few nutrients. In general, any nutritional deficiencies, whether of protein, energy or micronutrients, that are severe enough to lead to growth faltering are likely to result also in increased infection (Tomkins and Watson, 1989). The question remains whether more modest deficiencies of particular

nutrients impair infectious disease resistance and whether supplementation with these nutrients will reverse this impairment. Although many micronutrient deficiencies have been shown experimentally to impair immune functions and disease resistance in laboratory animals, this discussion will be limited to iron, zinc, and vitamin A, for which there is some evidence of clinical and public health importance.

Vitamin A is often deficient in weaning diets of children in poor families in developing countries. Infectious diseases such as measles (Reddy *et al.* 1986) and malaria (Thurnham and Singkamani, 1991) can further decrease vitamin A status as measured by plasma retinol levels. In less-developed countries, supplementation of young children with vitamin A decreases mortality and some indicators of severe morbidity (Beaton *et al.* 1993; Ghana VAST Study Team, 1993). However, supplementation, although potentially effective, should be viewed as only a short-term measure and efforts should be directed towards increasing the vitamin A content of weaning diets in areas where there is a high risk of vitamin A deficiency.

Zinc levels in weaning diets often exceed those in breast milk yet symptoms of zinc deficiency rarely show up before weaning, even in children suffering from genetic errors of zinc metabolism (Hambidge, 1986). It appears that the zinc in human milk is more readily absorbed and utilized than that from other diets. The zinc from diets that are predominantly vegetarian and high in fibre and phytates may be particularly unabsorbable (Forbes and Erdman, 1983). Zinc supplements have been shown to promote growth in children exhibiting failure to thrive after weaning (Hambidge, 1986). In Bangladeshi children with diarrhoea, zinc supplements for 2 weeks shortened the duration of illness and reduced the number of diarrhoeal episodes in the 2 months following discharge from hospital. The mechanism of this beneficial effect of zinc is unknown but may involve improvements in immune functions or changes in handling of water and electrolytes at the intestinal mucosa (S.K. Roy, A.M. Tomkins, R. Haider, R.H. Behrens, S.M. Akramuzzaman and D. Mahalanabis, unpublished results).

Considerable research has been conducted concerning interactions between infection and iron status. Iron deficiency impairs immune function and resistance to infection (Kuvibidila, 1987) and thus weaning diets need to provide adequate iron in a bioavailable form. Like zinc, iron from vegetable sources is relatively unavailable (Forbes and Erdman, 1983). Regular dietary iron is particularly important since attempts to replace iron stores rapidly by injection may have aggravated certain infections in adults and infants (Kuvibidila, 1987). Such large influxes of injected iron may overwhelm the homeostatic mechanisms that bind and sequester iron, reducing its plasma levels during infection (Kuvibidila, 1987).

Microbiological purity of weaning foods

Relatively little information is available concerning how to avoid microbial contamination of weaning foods in developing countries. It is generally unknown what proportion of infectious disease in infants is food-borne and what proportion comes from contaminated water, bottles and utensils or other objects in a generally poor or unhygienic environment. While the importance of clean water and hygiene should not be underplayed, in Nigeria it was found that installation of a drinking water and sanitation system had remarkably little effect on the morbidity from diarrhoea in infants (Huttly *et al.* 1990). Other research in which microbiological analysis of weaning foods was carried out suggests that these foods may be an important vector for infectious diseases (Black *et al.* 1989; Mensah *et al.* 1990). In poor families where fuel or maternal time is limited, weaning foods are likely to be prepared once a day rather than at every feeding (Tomkins, 1991). Particularly in countries where the ambient temperature is high, extensive growth of bacteria can occur between preparation and consumption of these foods (Mensah *et al.* 1990).

A scientifically neglected but traditionally common practice which appears to reduce microbial contamination of weaning foods is fermentation. In many cultures infants are traditionally given porridges or beverages made from fermented milk or grains (Tomkins *et al.* 1988). Maize that has been fermented according to Ghanaian practices has antimicrobial properties (Mensah *et al.* 1990). The low pH (<4.0) induced by the fermentation process is likely an important contributor to the inhibition of bacterial growth in fermented maize (Tomkins *et al.* 1988). In addition, there appears to be a heat-stable, ammonium sulphate-precipitable factor, possibly an antibiotic, which helps prevent microbial growth in fermented maize (Mensah *et al.* 1991). Further analysis of antimicrobial factors in fermented maize or other fermented cereals is warranted. More research is needed concerning possible adverse effects of these fermented foods on the infant's nutritional status and health before fermented weaning foods can be widely advocated. Nevertheless, where such foods are traditionally given to infants, this practice should be recognized as possibly beneficial and should not be discouraged, as has been done sometimes on the grounds that fermentation appears unhygienic.

CONCLUSIONS

The optimal infant feeding practices clearly depend greatly on the infant's environment. The evidence indicates that promotion of breast feeding in early infancy will benefit infants everywhere. In particular, the addition of potentially contaminated foods to the infant's diet should be delayed until

the infant's own defences have had a chance to mature, that is, until at least 4 months of age. Recent studies suggest a threshold over which further breast feeding appears to confer no additional resistance. A major thrust of research and public health programmes should be the provision of clean, safe, cheap, nutritionally adequate weaning foods in less-developed countries such that mothers have some decent options as to when and onto what foods they wean their children.

REFERENCES

Akre, J. (ed.) (1989) Infant feeding: the physiological basis. *WHO Bulletin OMS* (Suppl. 67), 1–108.

Andersson, B., Porras, O., Hanson, L.A. and Svanborg Eden, C. (1985) Non-antibody-containing fractions of breast milk inhibit epithelial attachment of *Streptococcus pneumoniae* and *Haemophilus influenzae*. *Lancet*, i, 643.

Bauchner, H., Leventhal, J.M. and Shapiro, E.D. (1986) Studies of breast-feeding and infections. How good is the evidence? *Journal of the American Medical Association*, **256**, 887–892.

Beaton, G.H., Martorell, R., L'Abbe, K.A. *et al.* (1993) *Effectiveness of Vitamin A Supplementation in the Control of Young Child Morbidity and Mortality in Developing Countries.* Toronto: CIDA.

Bertotto, A., Gerli, R., Fabietti, G. *et al.* (1990) Human breast milk T lymphocytes display the phenotype and functional characteristics of memory T cells. *European Journal of Immunology*, **20**, 1877–1880.

Black, R.E., de Romana, G.L., Brown, K.H. *et al.* (1989) Incidence and etiology of infantile diarrhea and major routes of transmission in Huascar, Peru. *American Journal of Epidemiology*, **129**, 785–799.

Blau, H., Paswell, J.H., Levanon, M. *et al.* (1983) Studies on human milk macrophages: effect of activation on phagocytosis and secretion of prostaglandin E2 and lysozyme. *Pediatric Research*, **17**, 241–245.

Brakohiapa, L.A., Bille, A., Quansah, E. *et al.* (1988) Does prolonged breastfeeding adversely affect a child's nutritional status? *Lancet*, ii, 416–418.

Brown, K.H., Black, R.E., de Romana, G.L. and de Kanashiro, H.C. (1989) Infant-feeding practices and their relationship with diarrheal and other diseases in Huascar (Lima), Peru. *Pediatrics*, **83**, 31–40.

Brown, K.H., Stallings, R.Y., de Kanashiro, H.C. *et al.* (1990) Effects of common illnesses on infants' energy intakes from breast milk and other foods during longitudinal community-based studies in Huascar (Lima), Peru. *American Journal of Clinical Nutrition*, **52**, 1005–1013.

Carpenter, G. (1980) Epidermal growth factor is a major growth-promoting agent in human milk. *Science*, **210**, 198–199.

Carver, J.D., Pimentel, B. and Barness, L.A. (1989) Nucleotide effects in formula-fed infants. *Pediatric Research*, **25**, 286A.

Carver, J.D., Pimentel, B., Wiener, D.A. *et al.* (1991) Infant feeding effects on flow cytometric analysis of blood. *Journal of Clinical Laboratory Analysis*, **5**, 54–56.

Chang, S. (1990) Antimicrobial proteins of maternal and cord sera and human milk in relation to maternal nutritional status. *American Journal of Clinical Nutrition*, **51**, 183–187.

Clemens, J., Rao, M., Ahmed, F. *et al.* (1993) Breast-feeding and the risk of life-threatening rotavirus diarrhea: prevention or postponement? *Pediatrics*, **92**, 680–685.

Coppa, G.V., Gabrielli, O., Giorgi, P. *et al.* (1990) Preliminary study of breast-feeding and bacterial adhesion to uroepithelial cells. *Lancet*, **335**, 569–571.

Crago, S.S., Prince, S.J., Pretlow, T.G. *et al.* (1979) Human colostral cells. 1. Separation and characterization. *Clinical and Experimental Immunology*, **38**, 585–597.

Cruz, J.R., Carlsson, B., Garcia, B. *et al.* (1982) Studies on human milk III. Secretory IgA quantity and antibody levels against *Escherichia coli* in colostrum and milk from underprivileged and privileged mothers. *Pediatric Research*, **16**, 272–276.

Davis, C.P., Houston, C.W., Fader, R.C. *et al.* (1982) Immunoglobulin A and secretory immunoglobulin A antibodies to purified type 1 *Klebsiella pneumoniae* pili in human colostrum. *Infection and Immunity*, **32**, 496–501.

Diaz-Jouanen, E. and Williams, R.C., Jr (1974) T and B lymphocytes in human colostrum. *Clinical Immunology and Immunopathology*, **3**, 248–255.

Duffy, L.C., Byers, T.E., Riepenhoff-Talty, M. *et al.* (1986) The effects of infant feeding on rotavirus-induced gastroenteritis: a prospective study. *American Journal of Public Health*, **76**, 259–263.

Editorial (1981) Microbial adhesion, colonisation, and virulence. *Lancet*, **ii**, 508–510.

Editorial (1988) Breast-feeding/breast milk and human immunodeficiency virus (HIV). *PAHO Bulletin*, **22**, 87–88.

Forbes, R. and Erdman, J.W., Jr (1983) Bioavailability of trace mineral elements. *Annual Review of Nutrition*, **3**, 213–231.

Gaull, G.E., Wright, C.E. and Isaacs, C.E. (1985) Significance of growth modulators in human milk. *Pediatrics*, **75**, 142–145.

Gendrel, D., Richard-Lenoble, D., Kombila, M. *et al.* (1989) Giardiasis and breast-feeding in urban Africa. *Pediatric Infectious Disease Journal*, **8**, 58–59.

Ghana VAST Study Team (1993) Vitamin A supplementation in northern Ghana: effects on clinic attendances, hospital admissions, and child mortality. *Lancet*, **342**, 7–12.

Gillin, F.D., Reiner, D.S. and Wang, C. (1983) Human milk kills parasitic intestinal protozoa. *Science*, **221**, 1290–1292.

Goldblum, R.M., Ahlstedt, S., Carlsson, B. *et al.* (1975) Antibody-forming cells in human colostrum after oral immunisation. *Nature*, **257**, 797–798.

Goldblum, R.M., Schanler, R.J., Garza, C. and Goldman, A.S. (1989) Human milk feeding enhances the urinary excretion of immunologic factors in low birth weight infants. *Pediatric Research*, **25**, 184–188.

Goldman, A.S., Garza, C., Nichols, B.L. and Goldblum, R.M. (1982) Immunologic factors in human milk during the first year of lactation. *Journal of Pediatrics*, **100**, 563–567.

Goldman, A.S., Thorpe, L.W., Goldblum, R.M. and Hanson, L.A. (1986) Anti-inflammatory properties of human milk. *Acta Paediatrica Scandinavica*, **75**, 689–695.

Gopalan, C. (1988) Stunting: significance and implications for public health policy. In *Linear Growth Retardation in Less Developed Countries*, pp. 265–284 (ed. J.C. Waterlow). New York: Raven Press.

Hambidge, K.M. (1986) Zinc deficiency in the weanling: how important? *Acta Paediatrica Scandinavica* (Suppl. 323), 52–58.

Hambraeus, L., Franson, G.T. and Lonnerdal, B. (1984) Nutritional availability of breast milk protein. *Lancet*, **ii**, 167–168.

Hennart, P.F., Brasseur, D.J., Delogne-Desnoeck, J.B. *et al.* (1991) Lysozyme, lactoferrin, and secretory immunoglobulin A content in breast milk: influence of duration of lactation, nutrition status, prolactin status, and parity of mother. *American Journal of Clinical Nutrition*, **53**, 32–39.

Herias, M.V., Cruz, J.R., Gonzalez-Cossio, T. *et al.* (1993) The effect of caloric supplementation on selected milk protective factors in undernourished Guatemalan mothers. *Pediatric Research*, **34**, 217–221.

Howie, P.W., Forsyth, J.S., Ogston, S.A *et al.* (1990) Protective effect of breast feeding against infection. *British Medical Journal*, **300**, 11–16.

Huttly, S.R.A., Blum, D., Kirkwood, B.R. *et al.* (1990) The Imo State (Nigeria) drinking water supply and sanitation project, 2. Impact on dracunculiasis, diarrhoea and nutritional status. *Transactions of the Royal Society of Tropical Medicine and Hygiene*, **84**, 316–321.

Jason, J.M., Nieburg, P. and Marks, J.S. (1984) Mortality and infectious disease associated with infant-feeding practices in developing countries. *Pediatrics* (Suppl.), 702–727.

Jelliffe, D.B. and Jelliffe, E.F.P. (1978) The volume and composition of human milk in poorly nourished communities: a review. *American Journal of Clinical Nutrition*, **31**, 492–515.

JHU/WHO (1989) Research on improving infant feeding practices to prevent diarrhoea or reduce its severity: memorandum from a JHU/WHO Meeting. *Bulletin of the World Health Organization*, **67**, 27–33.

Juto, P. (1985) Human milk stimulates B cell function. *Archives of Disease in Childhood*, **60**, 610–613.

Juto, P., Moller, C., Engberg, S. and Bjorksten, B. (1982) Influence of type of feeding on lymphocyte function and development of infantile allergy. *Clinical Allergy*, **12**, 409–416.

Keller, M.A., Kidd, R.M., Bryson, Y.J. *et al.* (1981) Lymphokine production by human milk lymphocytes. *Infection and Immunity*, **32**, 632–636.

Kuvibidila, S. (1987) Iron deficiency, cell-mediated immunity and resistance against infections: present knowledge and controversies. *Nutrition Research*, 7, 989–1003.

Lucas, A. (1986) Infant feeding. In *Textbook of Neonatology*, pp. 178–210 (ed. N.R.C. Roberton). Edinburgh: Churchill Livingstone.

Mensah, P.P.A., Tomkins, A.M., Drasar, B.S. and Harrison, T.J. (1990) Fermentation of cereals for reduction of bacterial contamination of weaning foods in Ghana. *Lancet*, **336**, 140–143.

Mensah, P., Tomkins, A.M., Drasar, B.S. and Harrison, T.J. (1991) Antimicrobial effect of fermented Ghanaian maize dough. *Journal of Applied Bacteriology*, **70**, 203–210.

Munoz, C., Endres, S., van der Meer, J. *et al.* (1990) Interleukin-1B in human colostrum. *Research in Immunology*, **141**, 505–513.

Narayanan, I., Prakash, K., Murthy, N.S. and Gujral, V.V. (1984) Randomised controlled trial of effect of raw and holder pasteurised human milk and of formula supplements on incidence of neonatal infection. *Lancet*, **ii**, 1111–1113.

Ogra, S.S. and Ogra, P.L. (1978) Immunologic aspects of human colostrum and milk. *Journal of Pediatrics*, **92**, 550–555.

Ostergaard, P.A.A. (1985) Serum and saliva Ig-levels in infants of non-atopic mothers fed breast milk or cow's milk-based formulas. *Acta Paediatrica Scandinavica*, **74**, 555–559.

Ozkaragoz, F., Rudloff, H.B., Rajaraman, S. *et al.* (1988) The motility of human milk macrophages in collagen gels. *Pediatric Research*, 23, 449–452.

Petschow, B.W. and Talbott, R.D. (1991) Response of *Bifidobacterium* species to growth promoters in human and cow milk. *Pediatric Research*, 29, 208–213.

Pittard, W.B., III and Bill, K. (1979) Immunoregulation by breast milk cells. *Cellular Immunology*, 42, 437–441.

Prentice, A. (1987) Breast feeding increases concentrations of IgA in infants' urine. *Archives of Disease in Childhood*, 62, 792–795.

Prentice, A., Prentice, A.M., Cole, T.J. and Whitehead, R.G. (1983) Determinants of variations in breast milk protective factor concentrations of rural Gambian mothers. *Archives of Disease in Childhood*, 58, 518–522.

Prentice, A., Ewing, G., Roberts, S.B. *et al.* (1987) The nutritional role of breast-milk IgA and lactoferrin. *Acta Paediatrica Scandinavica*, 76, 592–598.

Quan, R., Barness, L.A. and Uauy, R. (1990) Do infants need nucleotide supplemented formula for optimal nutrition? *Journal of Pediatric Gastroenterology and Nutrition*, 11, 429–437.

Reddy, V., Bhaskaram, P., Raghuramulu, N. *et al.* (1986) Relationship between measles, malnutrition, and blindness: a prospective study in Indian children. *American Journal of Clinical Nutrition*, 44, 924–930.

Roitt, I.M., Brostoff, J. and Male, D.K. (1989) *Immunology*. London: Gower Medical.

Sachdev, H.P.S., Krishna, J., Puri, R.K. *et al.* (1991) Water supplementation in exclusively breastfed infants during summer in the tropics. *Lancet*, 337, 929–933.

Saha, K., Garg, M., Rao, K.N. *et al.* (1987) Lymphocyte subsets in human colostrum with special reference to that of undernourished mothers. *Journal of Tropical Pediatrics*, 33, 329–332.

Schlesinger, J.J. and Covelli, H.D. (1977) Evidence for transmission of lymphocyte responses to tuberculin by breast-feeding. *Lancet*, ii, 529–532.

Stephens, S., Kennedy, C.R., Lakhani, P.K. and Brenner, M.K. (1984) In-vivo immune responses of breast- and bottle-fed infants to tetanus toxoid antigen and to normal gut flora. *Acta Paediatrica Scandinavica*, 73, 426–432.

Stephens, S., Brenner, M.K., Duffy, S.W. *et al.* (1986) The effect of breast-feeding on proliferation by infant lymphocytes in vitro. *Pediatric Research*, 20, 227–231.

Stoliar, O.A., Pelley, R.P., Kaniecki-Green, E. *et al.* (1976) Secretory IgA against enterotoxins in breast-milk. *Lancet*, i, 1258–1261.

Thurnham, D.I. and Singkamani, R. (1991) The acute phase response and vitamin A status in malaria. *Transactions of the Royal Society of Tropical Medicine and Hygiene*, 85, 194–199.

Tomkins, A. (1991) Recent developments in the nutritional management of diarrhoea. *Transactions of the Royal Society of Tropical Medicine and Hygiene*, 85, 4–7.

Tomkins, A., Alnwick, D. and Haggerty, P. (1988) Fermented foods for improving child feeding in eastern and southern Africa: a review. In *Improving Young Child Feeding in Eastern and Southern Africa*, (eds D. Alnwick, S. Moses and O.G. Schmidt) pp. 135–167. Ottawa: IDRC.

Tomkins, A. and Watson, F. (1989) *Malnutrition and Infection*. ACC/SCN, WHO, Geneva.

Underwood, B. A. (1985) Weaning practices in deprived environments: the weaning dilemma. *Pediatrics*, 75 (Suppl.), 194–198.

Victora, C.G., Vaughan, J.P., Martines, J.C. and Barcelos, L.B. (1984) Is prolonged breast-feeding associated with malnutrition? *American Journal of Clinical Nutrition*, 39, 307–314.

Victora, C.G., Vaughan, P., Lombardi, C. *et al.* (1987) Evidence for protection by breast-feeding against infant deaths from infectious diseases in Brazil. *Lancet*, **ii**, 319–321.

Viverge, D., Grimmonprez, L., Cassanas, G. *et al.* (1985) Variations of lactose and oligosaccharides in milk from women of blood types secretor A or H, secretor Lewis and Secretor H/non-secretor Lewis during the course of lactation. *Annals of Nutrition and Metabolism*, **29**, 1–11.

Walker, A.F. (1990) The contribution of weaning foods to protein–energy malnutrition. *Nutrition Research Reviews*, **3**, 25–47.

Walker, W.A. (1985) Absorption of protein and protein fragments in the developing intestine: role in immunologic/allergic reactions. *Pediatrics*, **75**, 167–171.

Weinberg, E.D. (1984) Iron withholding: a defense against infection and neoplasia. *Physiological Reviews*, **64**, 65–102.

Wright, A.L., Holberg, C.J., Martinez, F.D. *et al.* (1989) Breast feeding and lower respiratory tract illness in the first year of life. *British Medical Journal*, **299**, 946–949.

Zachman, R.D. (1989) Retinol (vitamin A) and the neonate: special problems of the human premature infant. *American Journal of Clinical Nutrition*, **50**, 413–424.

Ziegler, J.B. (1993) Breast feeding and HIV. *Lancet*, **342**, 1437–1438.

7

Use of cows' milk in infant feeding with emphasis on the compositional differences between human and cows' milk

Elizabeth M.E. Poskitt
MRC Dunn Nutrition Unit, Keneba, The Gambia

INTRODUCTION

Prior to 1974, and the first edition of the UK Department of Health publication *Present Day Practice in Infant Feeding* (DHSS, 1974), British infants who were not breast-fed were fed on cows' milk or formulas of reconstituted dried cows' milk. Feeds were prepared by adding slightly more water than had been removed in the drying process, and then sugar to increase the energy content. While the vast majority of infants thrived on these feeds, some developed serious complications and even died (Wharton, 1982). Since 1974 cows' milk and formulas of reconstituted unmodified cows' milk have not been recommended in Britain for infants under 6 months (DHSS, 1974). Scientific understanding of infant nutrition has increased greatly over the past 20 years and recommendations for the composition of infant formulas have expanded. Directives now regulate the composition and marketing of infant formulas and follow on formulas within the European Union.

The majority of medical and scientific personnel concerned with feeding human infants would agree that own mothers' milk is the ideal food for normal full-term infants. Nevertheless in many developed countries a significant proportion of newborn infants continue to be fed on infant formulas from birth. Many more will receive some formula when their mothers cease to breast feed at stages when the infants are not weaned or are still dependent on a liquid diet for a major proportion of their nutrient

Infant Nutrition. Edited by A.F. Walker and B.A. Rolls.
Published in 1994 by Chapman & Hall, London.
ISBN 0 412 59140 5.

needs. Manufacturers of infant formulas have been condemned widely for their marketing practices, especially in the developing world, but much of our nutritional understanding of the requirements of the newborn and of the uniqueness of human milk derives from close links between the nutritional scientists involved in commercial research and those involved in clinical research. Thus, while endorsing the superiority of human milk as food for infants, it is only realistic to encourage the development of safe preparations for feeding those infants who cannot receive maternal milk or whose mothers choose not to breast feed.

Traditionally, if infants are not fed on breast milk, they are given formula based on cows' milk. Although there has been an increase in the use of soya-based formulas for feeding infants, particularly when problems such as vomiting develop, the great majority of formula-fed infants continue to be fed on cows' milk-based formulas.

Why should neat cows' milk need modification before it is suitable for human infants? Simply, because it has evolved to feed calves, not humans. The composition of all mammalian milks varies (Widdowson, 1974). Differences in the major nutrients relate to differences in rates of growth, body composition (including the growth of hair, fur or horns), maturity at birth, and rates of postnatal maturation. Baby seals, for example, double their weight very rapidly after birth and deposit large amounts of subcutaneous fat but their mothers lactate for only short periods, secreting milk with a very high fat concentration and little lactose. Human milk has less fat and a much lower energy density, as befits a food for infants who take 4–5 months to double birth weight and who, in natural circumstances, are fed wholly on their mothers' milk for that length of time and, in part, for much longer.

It seems logical to concentrate discussion on those differences in composition between cows' and human milk that cause clinical problems when cows' milk is fed to young human infants. Many of these problems are now historical since cows' milk is no longer recommended for feeding young infants. The clinical problems that arose from now outdated feeding practices have determined some of the developments that have taken place in formula composition (DHSS, 1974; Schanler and Cheng, 1991). Thus, in discussing the problems of cows' milk for infants we shall also discuss the composition of modern formulas and how they compare with breast milk for nutrition of human infants.

COMPOSITION OF HUMAN AND COWS' MILK

Table 7.1 indicates concentrations of the major nutrients in cows' and human milk. Both milks, but particularly human milk, have tremendously varying composition, so the values given are approximations rather than

Table 7.1 Approximate composition of colostrum, mature human milk and cows' milk

	Colostrum	Human milk	Cows' milk
Energy			
(kJ/l)	[a]	2856	2730
(kcal/l)	[a]	680	650
Protein (g/l)	100	9	31
Casein (g/kg total protein)	160	300	800
Fat (g/l)	32	42	38
Polyunsaturated and monounsaturated fatty acids (g/kg total fatty acids)	590	470	250
Lactose (g/l)	53	70	49
Sodium (mM)	21	6.5	20
Chloride (mM)	17	12	30
Calcium (mM)	8	9	30
Phosphate (mM)	5	5	30
Calcium : phosphorus molar ratio	–	1.8	1.0
Iron (μM)	28	12.5	9.0
Vitamin A (μg/l)	1260	600	540
Vitamin C (mg/l)	70	38	10
Vitamin D (μg/l)	18	0.4	0.3

Compiled from Fomon (1974), Lucas (1986b), DHSS (1988), Williams (1991) and Hambraeus (1991).
[a]Energy content is difficult to determine since much of the protein is not absorbed.

precise values. The diversity of values given in reference texts shows the wide range of recorded values (Fomon, 1974; Jelliffe and Jelliffe, 1978; Lentner, 1981; Lucas, 1986b; George and de Francesca, 1989; Williams, 1991).

Differences between cows' and human milks in relation to the nitrogen content

Table 7.2 outlines differences in the quantity and quality of the various nitrogen-containing components of cows' and human milks.

The first milk produced in human lactation is colostrum. This is very different in composition from mature human milk as it has a high protein content (5–20 g secretory immunoglobulin A (sIgA)/l; 5 g lactoferrin/l) and high zinc and vitamin A concentrations. The composition of colostrum changes as lactation proceeds, so by 3 days of age milk is transitional, with composition between colostrum and mature human milk. Milk composition continues to change, albeit less dramatically, throughout the period of lactation.

Table 7.2 Approximate content of nitrogen sources in human and cows' milk

	Mature human milk	*Cows' milk*
Total protein (g/l)	9	31
Casein (g/kg total protein)	300	800
Whey proteins (g/l)		
α-Lactalbumin	3.6	2.3
β-Lactoglobulin	–	2.1
Lactoferrin	2.0	trace
Secretory IgA	0.8	trace
Amino acids (mg/l)		
Phenylalanine	400	1800
Phenylalanine : tyrosine ratio	1.3	1.0
Methionine	1200	800
Methionine : cysteine ratio	0.7	2.7
Non-protein nitrogen (mg/l)		
As mg/g total nitrogen	250	50
Urea	18	13
N-acetyl glucosamine	150	–
Free amino acids	50	48
Taurine	21.5	9.6
Taurine (mg/g total free amino acids)	430	20

Compiled from Fomon (1974), Lucas (1986b), Williams (1991) and Hambraeus (1991).

Protein

The protein concentration of cows' milk is more than three times that of mature human milk. Human colostrum has higher (100 g/l) protein content than mature human milk (DHSS, 1977) but much of the protein is in the form of sIgA which passes through the gut undigested and probably contributes little to nutrition (Jelliffe and Jelliffe, 1978).

Casein and whey

Milk proteins are divided into two groups: casein (curd) and whey proteins. Casein is that part of the milk precipitated at 20°C and acid pH 4.5. Whey protein is the protein that remains in the supernatant after extraction of casein (Schanler and Cheng, 1991). Cows' milk has a higher proportion of casein to whey proteins than human milk (casein content (g/l): cows', 800; human, 300) in addition to its higher total protein.

Casein is formed of various compounds bonded together into micellar formation as 'calcium caseinate complex' and associated phosphate, magnesium and citrate ions. Casein has a high proline content which may be responsible for the open structure of the molecules. Carboxypeptidase A

can digest the carboxyl terminals of amino acids in casein without disruption of the micellar structure and it is suggested that the spongy nature of the micellar structure allows free access of digestive enzymes into the centre of the micelles (George and de Francesca, 1989; Schanler and Cheng, 1991). The casein micelles of cows' milk are larger than those in human milk and form large flocculates in the upper bowel when fresh cows' milk is given to young infants (Jelliffe and Jelliffe, 1978; Hambraeus, 1991). Gastric emptying is delayed and, although this may facilitate digestion, if exaggerated it can lead to problems from tough agglomerated curds obstructing the intestinal lumen.

In the past, intestinal obstruction secondary to undigested casein curds obstructing the small intestine (lactobezoar or the inspissated curd syndrome) was not uncommon in young infants fed with neat cows' milk or unmodified cows' milk formulas. Modern cows' milk formulas have reduced total protein compared with cows' milk. Heat treatment in the course of preparation affects micellar formation so the curds, even in casein-predominant formulas, are less tough than in neat cows' milk. Young infants are able to digest the casein of modern formulas more readily. This, together with the greater use of whey-dominant formulas, makes intestinal obstruction less likely (Schreiner *et al*. 1982). Inspissated curd syndrome is still seen occasionally when curd-predominant formulas are given to infants with poor gastrointestinal function, particularly the premature (Schreiner *et al*. 1979).

Whey proteins form about 70% of the protein in human milk. Human and cows' milk whey proteins have different amino acid composition. Cows' milk-based formulas, in which the total protein and whey content have been modified to be quantitatively similar to human milk, still have very different overall amino acid composition when compared with human milk. Human milk whey protein consists mainly of α-lactalbumin, lactoferrin, sIgA and enzymes, especially lysozyme and bile salt-stimulated lipase. α-Lactalbumin binds calcium and may influence the bioavailability of calcium since calcium absorption is proportionately greater from human milk than from cows' milk (Charley and Slatman, 1953; Hambraeus, 1991).

The whey proteins of cows' milk are predominantly lactoglobulins. Since β-lactoglobulin is one of the proteins commonly responsible for cows' milk protein intolerance, there may be disadvantages in modifying the casein : whey ratios of cows' milk-based formulas so they are quantitatively similar to those of human milk. Cows' milk protein intolerance is more widely recognized than it used to be. It is not known whether this reflects a real increase in prevalence, perhaps due to higher concentrations of β-lactoglobulin in modern formulas, or simply better diagnosis of the problem.

Human milk contains proportionately much less methionine and more cysteine than cows' milk. The concentration of cysteine is approximately 250 mg/l in human milk compared with 130 mg/l in cows' milk. Methionine is the precursor of the sulphur-containing amino acid metabolic pathway. In adults cysteine is not an essential amino acid since it can be synthesized from methionine, although needs for methionine are reduced in the presence of adequate cysteine (Finkelstein and Mudd, 1967). Concentrations of cystathionase, the enzyme that catalyses the transsulphuration of methionine to cysteine, is low in the liver of the newborn. Thus there is potential cysteine deficiency, particularly amongst infants fed on cows' milk-based formulas without added cysteine and with premature infants, since liver cystathionase levels depend on maturity. After birth, irrespective of gestational age, cystathionase levels rise rapidly. Surprisingly, even those infants totally parenterally fed on cysteine-free infusions survive and thrive without added cysteine. Provided they receive sufficient methionine in their diet, young infants seem able to synthesize cysteine, perhaps outside the liver, in organs such as the kidneys, which have cystathionase activity (Zlotkin and Anderson, 1982).

The capacity both to synthesize and metabolize tyrosine shows limitations similar to those for cysteine. The newborn has about 60% of the adult activity of phenylalanine hydroxylase, which converts phenylalanine to tyrosine (Del Valle and Greengard, 1976). Infants fed with low-phenylalanine diets may be unable to synthesize sufficient tyrosine. When given high-tyrosine or high-phenylalanine diets, they may also have difficulty breaking down tyrosine to *p*-hydroxyphenyl pyruvic acid because tyrosine transaminase activity is only about 8% of adult levels. When neonates were fed with neat cows' milk and unmodified cows' milk formulas, transient hypertyrosinaemia and tyrosinuria were common findings, especially in the premature, because of this block in breakdown (Rassin, 1991). Inhibition of the next enzyme in the catabolic process – *p*-hydroxyphenylpyruvic acid oxidase – led to further hypertyrosinaemia. Transient tyrosinaemia could be distinguished from inborn errors of metabolism of the aromatic amino acids since tyrosine levels returned to normal with supplementary ascorbic acid. Ascorbic acid acted as a reducing agent and prevented inhibition of *p*-hydroxyphenylpyruvic acid oxidase, thus reducing the hypertyrosinaemia (Rassin *et al.* 1977).

Non-protein nitrogen

In addition to its constituent proteins, milk also contains non-protein nitrogen. This is present in the soluble, or whey, protein fraction of the

milk. It forms a small proportion of the total nitrogen in cows' milk but about 25% of the total nitrogen in human milk. In human milk most of the non-protein nitrogen is present as urea and free amino acids, especially glutamic acid and taurine.

The contribution of non-protein nitrogen to the nutrition of human infants is not entirely clear. The nitrogen content of human milk is low compared with most mammalian milks but infants utilize this nitrogen very efficiently. Blood urea levels in infants fed on human milk are much lower than those given either cows' milk or modern cows' milk-based formulas. The secretion of urea and/or the passage of non-protein nitrogen into the colon provides a source of nitrogen for amino acid synthesis by colonic bacteria. There is then the opportunity for reabsorption of urea nitrogen in a utilizable form (Heine *et al.* 1984; Millward *et al.* 1989). How much this occurs and how such recycling of nitrogen is regulated is unknown.

Taurine

Taurine is present in human milk in greater quantities than might seem necessary. Levels in cows' milk are very low (Rigo and Senterre, 1976; Rassin *et al.* 1978; Hayes, 1988). The relatively high levels of taurine in human milk remain unexplained. Taurine deficiency symptoms in full-term normal infants have not been described despite the fact that formula-fed infants were given taurine-free formulas for many years. Taurine-deficient kittens develop blindness, but there is no evidence in man that taurine deficiency is associated with problems in development of the eye or of vision – even in the premature (Jarvenpaa *et al.* 1983; Galeano *et al.* 1987).

Taurine is an important component of bile acids. Infants fed on low-taurine formula tend to conjugate bile acids with glycine rather than taurine. Although there is no discernible effect of a low-taurine diet on term infants and most studies have failed to show any evidence for clinical problems relating to taurine deficiency in prematures, one recent study does suggest that infants fed on taurine-deficient formulas have less efficient fat absorption (Galeano *et al.* 1987). This may result from the reduced stability of glycine-conjugated bile acids. Cystic fibrosis infants given low-taurine formulas also show poorer weight gain and more steatorrhoea (Darling *et al.* 1985; Thompson *et al.* 1987). Glycine-conjugated bile acids are readily precipitated in the acid pH of the duodenum in cystic fibrosis and are passively absorbed in the proximal rather than in the terminal ileum, leading to reduced efficiency of fat absorption.

Electrolytes and hyperosmolality problems

Renal solute load

The renal solute load includes those products from the digestion of food, largely nitrogenous waste products and electrolytes, that are not needed for growth and metabolism and must be excreted through the kidneys (Fomon, 1974). The high electrolyte content of cows' milk presents a dangerously high solute load to the kidneys of immature infants who can neither concentrate nor dilute their urine to the same capacity as older children. Dietary protein contributes to the renal solute load, particularly in infants fed cows' milk and high-protein unmodified cows' milk formulas. On cows' milk feeds a significant proportion of the electrolytes and the ingested and absorbed protein are not required as nitrogen for growth or metabolism and must be excreted. The practice in the 1960s and early 1970s of weaning from a few weeks of age on to high-protein, often salted, weaning foods increased the solute load further. Davies (1973) demonstrated that a high proportion of apparently normal, healthy, 6-week-old infants attending infant welfare clinics and being fed on unmodified cows' milk formulas had blood osmolality above the accepted normal range. Infants already on solids were even more likely to have abnormal plasma osmolality. The kidneys of these very young infants were failing to excrete the renal solute load derived from food. They were at great risk. Reduction in their fluid intakes due to anorexia with (for example) infection, increased extra renal loss of fluid with diarrhoea or pyrexia, or catabolism secondary to infection increasing nitrogenous breakdown products resulted in blood osmolalities rising to symptomatic levels. The initial high blood and extracellular fluid osmolality caused fluid to be drawn out of cells so there was intracellular dehydration and hyperosmolality. Ultimately renal loss of fluid to cope with the need to excrete sodium and urea led to extrarenal loss of fluid sufficient to cause circulatory collapse. The infants were usually in shock with renal, as well as pre-renal, failure. Plasma sodium and urea were grossly elevated. Vigorous resuscitation led to hyperosmolar cells mopping up intravenously administered fluids, which were iso-osmolar with normal plasma, too rapidly. Tissue distortion due to cellular overhydration, cerebral oedema, death or permanent brain damage were common results (Wharton, 1982).

Hypernatraemic dehydration in infancy has virtually disappeared owing to the modification of infant formulas and weaning solids. Modern cows' milk-based infant formulas have greatly reduced levels of protein and electrolytes. Cows' milk is no longer recommended for infants under 6 months of age and infant formulas or follow-on milks are preferable to cows' milk for infants under 1 year (DHSS, 1974, 1988).

Hypocalcaemia

All young infants have difficulty maintaining normal calcium levels. Hypocalcaemia is most common in the first 48 hours of life. Levels of calcium drop immediately after birth to reach their nadir around 24 hours of age. This drop is related to a number of factors. The high flux of calcium across the placenta from mother to fetus is cut off at birth. Calcium levels decline. At this early stage dietary calcium makes little contribution to the maintenance of normal serum calcium. As calcium levels fall, parathyroid hormone levels rise but so also do calcitonin levels (Pierson and Crawford, 1972). Calcitonin normally causes a fall in serum calcium by inhibition of bone resorption. It may be that the unexplained relative hypercalcitoninaemia of the newborn contributes to the fall in calcium, which is then exacerbated by a relative insensitivity to parathyroid hormone so the fall is not arrested.

Hypocalcaemia in neonates has rather different aetiologies depending on whether it occurs in the first half of the first week (early) or towards the end of the first week (late). Early neonatal hypocalcaemia is much more common in sick or immature neonates than in term infants and usually resolves in the first few days of life (Belton and Hambidge, 1991; Itani and Tsang, 1991). It probably has little to do with the type of feed an infant receives.

Late hypocalcaemia in otherwise normal newborns was common at the time infants were being fed on unmodified cows' milk formulas (Itani and Tsang, 1991). Cows' milk has a high phosphate content compared with human milk. Calcium is readily bound in the gut and absorption of phosphate occurs more readily than absorption of calcium. In the past, young infants fed on unmodified cows' milk formula occasionally developed hypocalcaemia with symptoms of tetany and convulsions around the sixth day of life (Brown *et al.* 1972; Pierson and Crawford, 1972). These infants fed well and absorbed phosphate at a greater rate than calcium. Phosphate levels in the blood rose and since calcium and phosphate levels interrelate, calcium levels fell and symptoms of hypocalcaemia developed. Relative unresponsiveness to parathyroid hormone contributed to the fall in serum calcium (Itani and Tsang, 1991).

There may be other factors than the phosphate intake involved in late hypocalcaemia since late neonatal hypocalcaemia is also associated with factors such as the time of year and maternal skin pigmentation, suggesting vitamin D metabolites are also relevant (Brown *et al.* 1972).

Treatment of late hypocalcaemia depended on giving intravenous calcium to elevate circulating calcium to asymptomatic levels and changing infants to low-phosphate formulas. Modern formulas have greatly reduced phosphate content as well as other electrolytes and in normal

Use of cows' milk in infant feeding

infants late hypocalcaemia secondary to the type of feed is now unusual (DHSS, 1974, 1988).

Carbohydrate

Lactose is the predominant carbohydrate in both human and cows' milks. The presence of lactose in milks facilitates calcium and magnesium absorption. Why this should be so is not entirely clear. It is possible lactose overcomes some metabolic block to calcium absorption (Wasserman, 1964). Alternatively, the relatively slow absorption of lactose leads to significant amounts of sugar in the lower small intestine, thus enhancing calcium absorption through the formation of calcium–lactose complexes which are more soluble than other calcium salts (Charley and Slatman, 1953).

For practical, often economic, reasons manufacturers have added a variety of carbohydrates to formulas as well as, or instead of, lactose. Glucose polymers – created by starch hydrolysis – are often used as they can maintain low formula osmolality at increased energy density. Glucose polymers are well tolerated by even pre-term infants and help stabilize formula composition. Table 7.3 lists the various polymer descriptions and their chain lengths.

The lactose content of human milk is higher than that of cows' milk. The lack of facilitated absorption of calcium with cows' milk may be overcome by the overall higher levels of calcium in cows' compared with human milk. Modern cows' milk-based formulas have added carbohydrate (which may or may not be lactose) to increase their energy content.

Other carbohydrates occurring naturally in milks are oligosaccharides, nucleotide sugars and lipid- and protein-bound carbohydrates. The non-lactose carbohydrates appear to be relevant to the typical *Bifidobacteria* and *Lactobacillus bifidus* flora in the colon of the breast-fed

Table 7.3 Chain length and description of glucose polymers used in infant formulas

Substance	Glucose units per molecule
Sugar	1–2
Glucose polymers	
Oligosaccharides	
Corn syrup	3–5
Maltodextrins	5–10
Polysaccharides	
Dextrins	10–20
Starch	20–2500

infant. Cows' milk-fed and formula-fed infants have predominantly Enterobacteriaeae in the colon. Human milk gangliosides also seem to include protective factors against *Vibrio cholerae* and *Escherichia coli* heat-labile toxin *in vitro*. The oligosaccharides of cows' milk are unlikely to mimic these effects.

Fats

As with other nutrients, there are both qualitative and quantitative differences in the fat content of human milk, cows' milk and cows' milk-based formulas. The qualitative differences are the most significant. Human milk contains not only C_{18} 'essential' fatty acids but also very long-chain (C_{20} and longer) polyunsaturated fatty acids (PUFA). The quantity of very long-chain PUFA in human milk is surprisingly constant compared with the variations in other components and is largely unaffected by dietary intakes. Cows' milk contains more saturated fat than human milk and less of the essential fatty acids linoleic ($18:2n–6$) and α-linolenic ($18:3n–3$) acids. It contains no C_{20} or longer-chain PUFA. Infants seem to thrive on cows' milk-based formulas that contain only the level of essential fatty acids in cows' milk, although plasma levels of C_{20} and C_{22} derivatives decline over time in those fed on cows' milk-based formulas. As well as being necessary for the developing brain, C_{20} and C_{22} PUFA are precursors of prostaglandins and leucotrienes involved in platelet adhesion and aggregation, vasoconstriction and many other physiological regulatory processes.

The brain can only utilize C_{20} and longer PUFA and these nutrients are structurally essential for normal brain and eye development. Other tissues can lengthen PUFA from linoleic and linolenic acids but there is concern that infants with limited energy and fat intakes (such as premature and/or growth-retarded neonates) may not be able to meet the very long-chain PUFA needs of the developing brain. FAO/WHO recommendations are that 3% of the energy in infant formulas should be from essential fatty acids and C_{20} and C_{22} derivatives should be included in formulas (Drury and Crawford, 1991). Moreover, since the $n–3$ and $n–6$ essential fatty acids compete for the 6-desaturase enzyme, the proportion of linoleic to α-linolenic acids has been recommended as between $5:1$ and $15:1$ (ESPGAN, 1991). Lucas *et al.* (1992) attribute better developmental outcome at 8-year follow-up in premature infants given some breast milk at birth, to the breast-fed infants' intakes of C_{20} and C_{22} PUFA. A study of the fatty acid composition of the brains of young infants dying suddenly and unexpectedly showed higher concentrations of docosahexaenoic ($22:6n–3$) acid in infants who had received breast milk than in those who received only cows' milk-based formula (Farquharson *et al.* 1992).

Further research is needed to establish the absolute requirements of young infants for individual very long-chain PUFA.

The fat content of modern formulas has been modified from cows' milk fats by the addition of vegetable oils. The proportions of saturated and unsaturated fatty acids present resemble those of human milk, but the actual fatty acids present are very different. Moreover, the fatty acid composition of human milks varies according to the prevailing fats in the mothers' diets.

Human milk has high levels of cholesterol (100–159 mg/l) and this has led to speculation that accustoming infants to high dietary cholesterol in early life equips them for metabolizing cholesterol efficiently, thus reducing the risks of hypercholesterolaemia and arteriosclerosis in later life. So far this concept remains interesting speculation only.

In addition to the high cholesterol content, human milk contains high levels of carnitine. Carnitine is absent from cows' milk and most cows' milk-derived formulas intended for normal term infants. Newborn infants can synthesize carnitine, but when growth and fat deposition are rapid it is possible that rates of endogenous carnitine synthesis limit rates of metabolism. External sources of carnitine may optimize growth rates in very young infants. Clinical effects have not been related to carnitine deficiency in normal full-term formula-fed infants but lack of dietary carnitine results in significantly lower levels of plasma carnitine in these infants (Hamosh, 1991).

Despite these differences in the fat of human and cows' milk, the main difference between the fat content of cows' and formula milks and that of human milk is the quantitative consistency of the former and the variation of the latter. Cows' milks as presented to the purchaser nowadays have fairly constant composition throughout the year. Formulas, if reconstituted correctly by mothers, also have constant composition. The fat in human milk varies in concentration according to the duration of lactation, the diet and nutritional state of the mother, the time of day and the stage of a feed. It has been suggested that the concentration of fat in the hindmilk (towards the end of a feed) provides satiety. This helps infants develop appetite regulation and prevents later obesity. This again would be an interesting phenomenon if it were supported by evidence that breast feeding is protective against obesity. However, evidence that infants stop feeding because of the high fat content at the end of a feed is not strong and may be difficult to equate with diurnal variations in milk fat concentrations.

Saturated fats tend to be less well absorbed than unsaturated fats. Newborn infants only absorb about 65% of the fat in cows' milk compared with 95% of the fat in human milk. Absorption from modern formulas is closer to that of human milk than of cows' milk. Saturated fats

also bind with electrolytes in the gut to form insoluble soaps which then bind calcium and other minerals in the gut as well.

In human milk the saturated fatty acids, particularly palmitic acid, tend to be positioned on the second arm of the glycerol molecule. Digestion of peripheral fatty acids from triacylglycerols leaves monoacylglycerols bearing the saturated fatty acids. Absorption of saturated fatty acid monoacylglycerols is more efficient than that of free saturated fatty acids. If palmitic acid is bound as a monoacylglycerol there is also less free palmitic acid available in the gut to bind with calcium and magnesium to form insoluble soaps. Thus the position of the fatty acids on the triacylglycerol molecule can be important in the efficiency of absorption of both fats and minerals (Fomon, 1974).

Lipase and fat absorption

Of the energy from breast milk or formula, 40–50% comes from fat. Since energy needs in infancy are high and in the very young infant as much as 30% of energy intake is required for growth, efficient fat absorption is important in infancy (Widdowson, 1974). In older children and adults fats are hydrolysed by the action of pancreatic lipases and then solubilized by bile salt action prior to absorption. Pancreatic and hepatic functions are not fully developed in the newborn and pancreatic lipase and bile salt concentrations in the gut are low.

Fat droplets in milk are coated with phospholipids and proteins, which might seem to protect them from fat digestion. Fat digestion and absorption in young infants are enhanced by the action of lingual lipases. These are secreted by papillae on the posterior part of the tongue and have the capacity to penetrate the fat particles and hydrolyse triacylglycerols without disrupting the fat globule membrane. Lingual lipase hydrolyses medium-chain and short-chain triacylglycerols very rapidly and the monoacylglycerols so formed are absorbed directly through the gastric mucosa and appear rapidly in the circulation. The monoacylglycerols and fatty acids also help emulsify the remaining fat, thus compensating for low bile salt content. In formula-fed infants lingual lipases are the main agents of lipolysis. Breast milk contains a bile salt-stimulated lipase which also facilitates digestion and absorption of fats and probably accounts for their better absorption from human milk than from cows' milk-based formulas.

Vitamin and mineral content

Modern British infant formulas all have added vitamins and minerals. The vitamin C and D content of cows' milk is very dependent on the time of year and whether the cows have been eating fresh grass. The iron content of both cows' and human milk is low. In human milk, lactoferrin

facilitates absorption of iron by its iron-binding capacity. The low vitamin C and D and particularly the low iron content of cows' milk has led to the recommendation that mothers keep their infants on breast milk, infant or follow-on formula until 1 year of age rather than change to cows' milk at 6 months, as had been suggested previously (DHSS, 1988).

Iron

The absorption of iron from human milk is much higher (45–75%) than from cows' milk (10%) or supplemented formula (7–8%) (Lonnerdal, 1984). This has been attributed to the high lactoferrin content of human milk and its absence from cows' milk and infant formulas (Brock, 1980). Lactoferrin binds specifically to a receptor in the brush border membrane of the small intestine and this may account for the high bioavailability of lactoferrin-bound iron (Hambraeus, 1991). However, it now seems that only 30–40% of iron is associated with lactoferrin. About 33% of iron is found in the fat portion of milk, bound to xanthine oxidase, in the outer fat globule membrane. The relationship of lactoferrin and its binding capacity and the facilitated absorption of iron in human milk remains unclear (Lonnerdal, 1984; Hambraeus, 1991).

Infants are born with a relatively high blood haemoglobin (180–200 g/l). Acceptable haemoglobin levels for infants after the first months of life and in early childhood are lower (100–120 g/l) than for adults. Since most of the iron in the body is contained in haemoglobin and there is relatively little iron in human breast milk, breast-fed infants need an external source of iron around the age at which they double their birth weights, since by then they will also have doubled their blood volumes. This is one of the reasons for recommending weaning at 4–5 months (Dallman, 1986). Weaning is a gradual process, however, and it may be some months before infants are receiving adequate nutrients from foods other than milk. Milk still forms a major component of the diet of most children at 1 year. Thus early introduction to a low-iron milk – cows' milk – is a risk factor for later iron deficiency.

Zinc

Better absorption of zinc in human milk has interesting significance for the rare condition of acrodermatitis enteropathica. Here there is a defect in zinc absorption which leads to symptoms of zinc deficiency with failure to thrive, mucocutaneous ulceration and ultimately death. Breast-fed infants with acrodermatitis enteropathica usually only develop symptoms when weaned. Those fed on cows' milk-based formulas develop symptoms and signs much earlier. The condition is prevented by zinc supplementation (Barnes and Moynahan, 1973).

Vitamin E

Newborn infants have low circulating levels of vitamin E. Levels rise in the first 2 weeks of life in breast-fed infants. They remain low in premature infants. Vitamin E is important as a lipid antioxidant which scavenges free radical intermediaries which may otherwise peroxidize polyunsaturated fatty acids and disrupt the architecture of cell membranes. Needs for vitamin E are related to the polyunsaturated fatty acid content of the diet. This relationship was first shown in the newborn when infant formulas with high polyunsaturated fatty acids content were introduced many years ago in the USA. Many infants on these formulas developed haemolytic anaemias which were prevented or treated by vitamin E supplementation. Since then vitamin E has been added to formulas containing polyunsaturated fatty acids in excess of cows' milk fat. Recommendations are that milks contain α-tocopherol in amounts not less than 0.4 mg α-tocopherol to 1 g polyunsaturated fatty acids (DHSS, 1980).

Vitamin K

One of the main nutritional problems seen in infants fed on human milk and given no protective supplementation is haemorrhagic disease of the newborn resulting from vitamin K deficiency. Human milk has low vitamin K content. Newborn infants are born with low vitamin K levels (Schwarz, 1989). Modern formulas have added vitamin K and cows' milk has a higher concentration of vitamin K than human milk, so the problem was seen less commonly, even before supplementation of formulas, in artificially fed infants. Intramuscular 1 mg vitamin K at birth effectively prevents haemorrhagic disease in normal term infants. Oral vitamin K is effective with most breast-fed infants but occasional infants seem to require more than one dose to counteract any bleeding tendencies. Recommendations are that formulas should contain at least 15 μg/l vitamin K (DHSS, 1980).

Non-nutritional factors of significance in human milk and not present in formula milk

While modern infant cows' milk-based formulas resemble human milk in many *quantitative* aspects, they remain different from human milk in many important *qualitative* aspects. Currently manufacturers of infant formulas are unable to correct all these qualitative differences although this may be possible in the near future.

Table 7.4 lists some of the anti-infective properties of human milk (see also Walker and Hong, 1973). These factors are discussed elsewhere in this book. Some have nutritional as well as immunological effects. Thus

Table 7.4 Anti-infective properties of human milk

Cellular
  Lymphocytes
  Neutrophils
  Macrophages
Humoral
  Proteins
    Secretory immunoglobulin A
    Lactoferrin
    Other nutrient-binding proteins
    Lysozyme
    Peroxidase
    Bile salt-stimulated lipase
  Complement
  Interferon
  Oligosaccharides
  Bifidus factor: nitrogen-containing polysaccharide
  High polyunsaturated fatty acid concentration
  Low buffering capacity

lactoferrin facilitates the absorption of iron and this prevents the use of iron by bacteria for multiplication. Similar ligands and proteins in human milk bind and facilitate absorption of folate, cyanocobalamin (vitamin B_{12}) and zinc as well as other minerals and vitamins. These may also have protective effects against infection.

Human milk is a vehicle for enzymes and hormones. The real role of many of these is not established but some have significance for infant feeding (Lucas, 1986a).

Human milk contains glucuronidase. This enzyme breaks down conjugated bilirubin secreted into the gut down the bile duct, allowing bilirubin to be reabsorbed. Liver function in the newborn is immature and has difficulty conjugating the load of bilirubin presented from red cell breakdown. High glucuronidase activity in some breast milks leads to the liver being presented with an extra load of reabsorbed bilirubin. The 'breast milk jaundice' that develops in some thriving breast-fed infants at the end of the first week of life and persisting for several weeks probably relates to high breast milk glucuronidase levels (Gourlay and Arend, 1986).

WHAT IS THE PLACE FOR COWS' MILK IN INFANT FEEDING?

Neat cows' milk is not recommended for infants under 6 months in Britain (DHSS, 1988) and the most recent recommendations are that

mothers should not give cows' milk feeds to infants under 12 months of age. In early infancy the main disadvantage of cows' milk is the high electrolyte and protein load. In later infancy the low iron and vitamin levels make cows' milk unsuitable for infants who are not yet on full weaning diets. Infant formulas, which in Britain are supplemented with iron and vitamins A, C and D, should be used instead of cows' milk, if the infants are not still breast-fed, until 1 year. There is a choice between casein- and whey-based formulas, cows' milk protein- and soya protein-based formulas and, after 6 months, between infant formulas and the follow-on formulas that are intended for infants taking formulas as part of weaning diets.

The modifications needed to make cows' milk a suitable diet for young infants have been alluded to earlier in this chapter. Table 7.5 indicates some of the modifications that characterize particular brands of milk, although manufacturers change feed composition from time to time and the composition of the formulas indicated here may have only transient value.

MODERN INFANT FORMULAS

The characteristics of some cows' milk-based infant formulas outlined in Table 7.5 show that there is a wide range of formulas with slightly different composition. However, there is little evidence that any one is better than the others for normal-term infants. It seems sensible that those that most resemble human milk in composition should be recommended for newborn infants. Many mothers like to feel their infants are growing up and demonstrate this by changing the formulas because their first choices of formula 'do not satisfy' their infants. There seems little evidence that 'satisfaction' is any greater with one formula compared with others and these differences are subjective impressions of mothers rather than objective clinical findings.

HOW ARE MODERN INFANT FORMULAS ADAPTED?

All modern formulas have reduced protein and reduced electrolytes compared with cows' milk and added iron and vitamins A, B group, C, D, E and K. They now also have added taurine and some have added carnitine.

In some, the predominant proteins are caseins and in some the protein has been supplemented with demineralized whey so there is a higher proportion of whey proteins. Because the amino acid content of cows' milk protein, whether casein or whey, is not the same as that in human milk, the protein content needs to be slightly higher than in human milk. In whey protein-dominant formulas, protein levels need not be as high as

Table 7.5 Approximate composition of some infant formulas available in the UK

Formula	Energy (MJ/l)	Protein	Carbo-hydrate (g/l)	Fat	Na	Cl	Ca (mg/l)	P	Sources[a] of: Carbo-hydrate	Fat
Highly modified formulas: whey > casein; PUFA > SFA										
Gold (Wyeth)	2.72	15	70	36	150	400	420	280	L	V
Premium (C&G)	2.85	14	73	36	180	400	540	270	L	VB
Ostermilk I (Crookes)	2.72	15	70	38	190	310	350	450	D	VB
Aptamil (Milupa)	2.80	15	72	36	180	380	590	180	L	VB
Less highly modified casein > whey; variable fats										
White (Wyeth)	2.72	15	72	36	180	420	460	360	L	VA
Plus (C&G)	2.76	19	73	34	250	600	850	520	L	VB
Ostermilk II (Crookes)	2.72	17	86	26	250	310	610	490	LD	V
Milumil (Milupa)	2.85	19	84	31	240	270	710	550	LD Am	VB
Follow-on formulas										
Progress (Wyeth)	2.72	29	80	26	350	750	1150	940	LG	V
Junior	2.80	20	80	30	300	650	720	590	DA	VB

[a]Abbreviations: A, animal fats; Am, amylose; B, full cream milk, butterfat; D, maltodextrins; G, glucose syrup; L, lactose; V, vegetable oils; C&G, Cow & Gate.

in casein-dominant formulas since the amino acid patterns are closer to those of human milk. Recommendations are that the amount of protein (total N × 6.38) in milks with the casein : whey ratio of cows' milk should be at least 15 g/l but not more than 20 g/l of reconstituted feed. Formulas with a casein : whey ratio close to that characteristic of human milk may have lower protein but total protein should still be at least 12 g/l (DHSS, 1980).

The fats of cows' milk formulas are either butterfats (beef fats have been used) or mixtures of vegetable oils. Vegetable oil mixtures have higher polyunsaturated fatty acid content than butterfats. They are often closer to the pattern of saturation of fatty acids in human milk but the actual fatty acids remain very different.

In addition to the standard formulas for normal healthy term infants there are two other types of infant cows' milk-based formulas. Premature

infants have particular needs in terms of energy, protein, minerals and vit-amins and these are not adequately met by modern term infant formulas. Thus a group of formulas for pre-term low-weight infants (usually reserved for those under 2 kg) have been developed. At the other end of the infant feeding spectrum are infants who would have changed to cows' milk at 6 months. The low iron and vitamin content of cows' milk makes it unsuitable for young weanlings. Yet many mothers seem reluctant to continue to feed standard formula – they want their babies to grow up. 'Follow-on' milks have developed to meet the needs of the older infants. These are formulas with higher electrolyte, iron and protein concentration since they are perceived as meeting the needs of infants who are receiving some weaning solids which will contribute to energy intakes so the infants will ingest (per kilogram body weight) volumes of milk lower than for those on formula only. Thus essential nutrients are supplied in smaller volumes. The age at which follow-on formulas should be recommended is controversial. Recommendations in Britain are that follow-on formulas are not used before 6 months of age. EC directives appear to accept their use from 4 months onwards. The controversy lies probably more in what policy provides safe population guidelines, rather than what is actually safe in individuals.

Recommendations that these feeds are safe for infants at 4 months means that some infants are likely to receive them much younger. The high sodium and protein content carries a significant risk to very young infants. Currently, however, follow-on milks are not used very much in the UK. Their popularity in Continental Europe may relate to the lower volumes of milk drunk by older children and adults and to the absence of a daily doorstep milk delivery. A direct move from breast feeding or infant formula to cows' milk at 1 year would seem closer to the traditional progression for feeding British infants.

Low birth weight infants show better weight gain, greater nitrogen absorption and nitrogen retention and decreased urea production on whey-dominant cows' milk formulas than on casein-dominant formulas. This is presumably due to more appropriate balance of amino acids for human growth and metabolism. In mature human infants there is no evidence of better nitrogen retention, although the plasma amino acid profiles of infants on whey-dominant formulas are closer to those of full-term infants fed human milk.

Since the introduction of protein-reduced cows' milk formulas and the greater use of whey-predominant formulas in Britain in the mid-1970s, patterns of early infant growth have changed. Infants put on weight less rapidly and seem less obese. However, a number of changes in infant feed-ing practices occurred at the same time as the protein content of formula was reduced. Changes in growth may have related more to reductions in

the volumes of formula ingested and to delays in the introduction of weaning solids than to changes in the quantity or quality of protein in the formulas.

HOW WILL FORMULAS CHANGE IN THE FUTURE?

Despite their superficial resemblances to human milk, modern formulas still lack many factors present in human milks, although the role of most of these factors may be more physiological than nutritional. Table 7.6 lists factors in human milk that are currently unreplicated in formula. Although it is desirable that some of these factors should be incorporated into formula, it is likely that it will not be practical, possible or even desirable to introduce all (Goldman and Garza, 1987). One manufacturer has already introduced arachidonic (20:4n–6) and docosahexaenoic acids into a commercial product for premature infants. However, potential problems with stability and possible contaminants of very long-chain PUFA may delay further PUFA additions to formula until there has been more research. Some anti-infective humoral factors, as opposed to cellular factors, are also potential additions to formula. There is currently research on introducing some form of lactoferrin into formulas.

It is likely that formula composition will continue to be modified and adapted with progress in scientific skills and nutritional understanding. Nevertheless, for the normal healthy full-term infant it is unlikely that the composition of infant formulas will ever provide the variety of nutrient and active factors provided by maternal milk. And it is highly unlikely that formula will ever reproduce the individuality or the changing composition of own mother's milk which uniquely caters for the changing needs of her growing, maturing infant.

Table 7.6 Factors present in human milk that may have nutritional value and are currently not present in standard infant formulas

Carnitine
Cholesterol
Nucleotides
Polyamines
Long-chain polyunsaturated fatty acids
Non-protein nitrogen
Urea
Free amino acids
Glycosamine
Enzymes, especially bile salt-stimulated lipase

REFERENCES

Barnes, P.M. and Moynahan, E.J. (1973) Zinc deficiency in acrodermatitis enteropathica: multiple dietary imbalances treated with synthetic diet. *Proceedings of the Royal Society of Medicine*, **66**, 327–329.

Belton, N.R. and Hambidge, K.M. (1991) Essential element deficiency and toxicity. In *Textbook of Paediatric Nutrition*, 3rd edn, pp. 429–451 (eds D.S. McLaren, D. Burman, N.R. Belton and A.F. Williams). Edinburgh: Churchill Livingstone.

Brock, J.H. (1980) Lactoferrin in human milk: its role in iron absorption and protection against enteric infection in the newborn infant. *Archives of Disease in Childhood*, **55**, 417–421.

Brown, J.K., Cockburn, F. and Forfar, J.O. (1972) Clinical and chemical correlates in convulsions in the newborn. *Lancet*, **i**, 135–139.

Charley, P. and Slatman, P. (1953) Chelation of calcium by lactose: its role in transport mechanisms. *Science*, **139**, 1205–1206.

Dallman, P.R. (1986) Iron deficiency in the weanling: a nutritional problem on the way to resolution. *Acta Paediatrica Scandinavica* (Supp. 323), 59–67.

Darling, P.B., Lepage, G., Leroy, C. *et al.* (1985) Effect of taurine supplement on fat absorption in cystic fibrosis. *Pediatric Research*, **19**, 578–585.

Davies, D.P. (1973) Plasma osmolality and feeding practices of healthy infants in the first three months of life. *British Medical Journal*, **2**, 340–342.

Del Valle, J.A. and Greengard, O. (1976) Phenylalanine hydroxylase and tyrosine aminotransferase in human fetal and adult liver. *Pediatric Research*, **11**, 2–5.

DHSS (Department of Health and Social Security) (1974) *Present Day Practice in Infant Feeding*. Reports on Health and Social Subjects no. 9. London: HMSO.

DHSS (Department of Health and Social Security) (1977) *The Composition of Mature Human Milk*. Reports on Health and Social Studies no. 12. London: HMSO.

DHSS (Department of Health and Social Security) (1980) *Artificial Feeds for the Young Infant*. Reports on Health and Social Subjects no. 18. London: HMSO.

DHSS (Department of Health and Social Security) (1988) *Present Day Practice in Infant Feeding: Third Report*. Reports on Health and Social Subjects no. 32. London: HMSO.

Drury, P.J. and Crawford, M.A. (1991) Essential fatty acids in human milk. In *Clinical Nutrition in the Young Child*, pp. 302–312 (eds O. Brunser, F.R. Carrazza, M. Gracey, B.L. Nichols and J. Senterre). New York: Raven Press.

ESPGAN (1991) Committee on Nutrition. Comment on the content and composition of lipid in infant formula. *Acta Paediatrica Scandinavica*, **80**, 887–896.

Farquharson, J., Cockburn, F., Patrick, W.A. *et al.* (1992) Infant cerebral cortex phospholipid fatty-acid composition and diet. *Lancet*, **340**, 810–813.

Finkelstein, J.D. and Mudd, S.H. (1967) Transsulfuration in mammals: the methionine sparing effect of cysteine. *Journal of Biological Chemistry*, **242**, 873–880.

Fomon, S.J. (1974) *Infant Nutrition*. Philadelphia, PA: W. B. Saunders.

Galeano, N.F., Darling, P., Lepage, G. *et al.* (1987) Taurine supplementation of a premature formula improves fat absorption in preterm infants. *Pediatric Research*, **22**, 67–71.

George, D.E. and de Francesca, B.A. (1989) Human milk in comparison to cow milk. In *Textbook of Gastroenterology and Nutrition in Infancy*, 2nd edn, pp. 243–264 (ed. E. Lebenthal). New York: Raven Press.

Goldman, A.S. and Garza, C. (1987) Future research in human milk. *Pediatric Research*, 22, 493–496.

Gourlay, G.R. and Arend, R.A. (1986) β-Glucuronidase and hyperbilirubinaemia in breast fed and formula fed babies. *Lancet*, i, 644–646.

Hambraeus, L. (1991) Human milk: nutritional aspects, part I. In *Clinical Nutrition of the Young Child*, pp. 289–301 (eds O. Brunser, F.R. Carrazza, M. Gracey, B.L. Nichols and J. Senterre). New York: Raven Press.

Hamosh, M. (1991) Lipid metabolism. In *Neonatal Nutrition and Metabolism*, pp. 122–142 (ed. W.W. Hay). St Louis, MO: Mosby Year Books.

Hayes, K.C. (1988) Taurine nutrition. *Nutrition Research Reviews*, 1, 99–113.

Heine, W., Tiess, M., Stolpe, H.J. and Wutzke, K.D. (1984) Urea utilization by the intestinal flora of infants fed mothers' milk and formula diet as measured with a ^{15}N tracer technique. *Journal of Pediatric Gastroenterology and Nutrition*, 3, 709–712.

Itani, O. and Tsang, R.C. (1991) Calcium, phosphate and magnesium in the newborn: pathophysiology and management. In *Neonatal Nutrition and Metabolism*, pp. 171–202 (ed. W.W. Hay). St Louis, MO: Mosby Year Books.

Jarvenpaa, A.L., Raiha, N.C.R., Rassin, D.K. and Gaull, G.E. (1983) Feeding the low birth weight infant. I. Taurine and cholesterol supplementation of formula does not affect growth and metabolism. *Pediatrics*, 71, 171–178.

Jelliffe, D.B. and Jelliffe, E.F.P. (1978) *Human Milk in the Modern World*. Oxford: Oxford University Press.

Lentner, C. (1981) *Geigy Scientific Tables: Units of Measurement, Body Fluids, Composition of the Body, Nutrition*, 8th edn, vol. 1, p. 214. Basle: Ciba-Geigy.

Lonnerdal, B. (1984) Iron and breast milk. In *Iron Nutrition in Infancy and Childhood*, pp. 95–117 (ed. A. Stekel). New York: Raven Press.

Lucas, A. (1986a) Infant feeding. In *Textbook of Neonatology*, pp. 178–192 (ed. N.R.C. Roberton). Edinburgh: Churchill Livingstone.

Lucas, A. (1986b) Feeding the full term infant. In *Textbook of Neonatology*, pp. 193–203 (ed. N. R. C. Roberton). Edinburgh: Churchill Livingstone.

Lucas, A., Morley, R., Cole, T.J. *et al.* (1992) Breast milk and subsequent intelligence quotient in children born pre-term. *Lancet*, 339, 261–264.

Millward, D.J., Jackson, A.A., Price, G. and Rivers, J.P.W. (1989) Human amino acid and protein requirements: current dilemmas and uncertainties. *Nutrition Research Reviews*, 2, 109–132.

Pierson, J.D. and Crawford, J.D. (1972) Dietary dependent neonatal hypocalcemia. *American Journal of Diseases of Children*, 123, 472–474.

Rassin, D.K. (1991) Aminoacid and protein metabolism in the premature and term infant. In *Neonatal Nutrition and Metabolism*, pp. 110–121 (ed. W.W. Hay). St Louis, MO: Mosby Year Books.

Rassin, D.K., Gaull, G.E. and Raiha N.C.R. (1977) Milk protein quantity and milk protein quality in low birth weight infants. 4. Effects on tyrosine and phenylalanine in plasma and urine. *Journal of Pediatrics*, 90, 356–360.

Rassin, D.K., Sturman, J.A. and Gaull, G.E. (1978) Taurine and other free aminoacids in milk of man and other mammals. *Early Human Development*, 2, 1–13.

Rigo, J. and Senterre, J. (1976) Is taurine essential in the milk of man and other mammals? *Biology of the Neonate*, 32, 73–76.

Schanler, R.J. and Cheng, S.-F. (1991) Infant formulas for enteral feeding. In *Neonatal Nutrition and Metabolism*, pp. 303–334 (ed. W.W. Hay). St Louis, MO: Mosby Year Books

Schreiner, R.L., Brady, M.S., Franken, E.A. *et al.* (1979) Increased incidence of lactobezoars in low birth weight infants. *American Journal of Diseases of Children*, **133**, 936–940.

Schreiner, R.L., Brady, M.S., Ernst, J.A. and Lemoine, J.A. (1982) Lack of lactobezoars in infants given predominantly whey formulas. *American Journal of Diseases of Children*, **136**, 437–439.

Schwarz, K.B. (1989) Requirements and absorption of fat soluble vitamins during infancy. In *Textbook of Gastroenterology and Nutrition in Infancy*, 2nd edn, pp. 347–366 (ed. E. Lebenthal). New York: Raven Press.

Thompson, G.N., Robb, T.A. and Davidson, G.P. (1987) Taurine supplementation, fat absorption and growth in cystic fibrosis. *Journal of Pediatrics*, **111**, 501–506.

Walker, W.A. and Hong, R. (1973) Immunology of the gastrointestinal tract. Part I. *Journal of Pediatrics*, **83**, 517–530.

Wasserman, R.H. (1964) Lactose stimulates gastrointestinal absorption of calcium: theory. *Nature*, **139**, 997–999.

Wharton, B,A. (1982) Food for the suckling: evolution and development. *Acta Paediatrica Scandinavica* (Suppl.), **299**, 5–10.

Widdowson, E.M. (1974) Nutrition. In *Scientific Foundations of Paediatrics*, pp. 41–53 (eds J.A. Davis and J.Dobbing). London: Heinemann.

Williams, A.F. (1991) Lactation and infant feeding. In *Textbook of Paediatric Nutrition*, 3rd edn, pp. 21–46 (eds D.S. McLaren, D. Burman, N.R. Belton and A.F. Williams). Edinburgh: Churchill Livingstone.

Zlotkin, S.H. and Anderson, G.H. (1982) The development of cystathionase activity during the first year of life. *Pediatric Research*, **16**, 65–68.

8
Food allergy and intolerance in infancy

D. Anne Moneret-Vautrin

Immunologie Clinique et Allergologie, Hôpital de Brabois,
Vandoeuvre-les-Nancy, France

INTRODUCTION

Food allergy and pseudoallergic reactions to food

Food allergy includes all the clinical manifestations associated with an immunological mechanism, that is, with a sensitization to food allergens or trophallergens, mediated by specific immunoglobulin E (IgE). These allergens are proteins, most often of average molecular mass between 20 and 60 kDa (Bleumink, 1970; Moneret-Vautrin, 1986).

Contact with trophallergens occurs early: at birth as far as cows' milk proteins are concerned if the child is not breast-fed, and at 3–6 months for other foods. Even in the case of breast-fed children, contact with food proteins takes place at birth, since the mother's milk contains them. Further, these proteins undeniably cross the placental barrier (Warner, 1980), and exceptional cases of *in utero* sensitization have been described (Matsumura and Kuroume, 1975). Consequently, allergic reactions may occur on the first known exposure to the food (Van Asperen *et al.* 1983).

This is why food allergy is the first sign of atopy in children who are genetically predisposed to synthesizing specific IgE against environmental allergens. It has been shown that babies with high rates of specific IgE to egg white at the age of 8 months all develop respiratory allergies in the 7 years following (Hattevig *et al.* 1987).

The physiopathology of IgE-dependent allergy is well known. IgE

Infant Nutrition. Edited by A.F. Walker and B.A. Rolls.
Published in 1994 by Chapman & Hall, London.
ISBN 0 412 59140 5.

antibodies attach to cells on membrane receptors of high affinity (for mast cells and basophils) and of low affinity (for B-lymphocytes, monocytes, macrophages and Langerhans cells). The binding of two specific IgE molecules by the allergen on the mast cells and basophils triggers the release of chemical mediators, principally histamine. Histamine produces pharmacological effects: vasodilatation, hyperpermeability, contraction of unstriated muscle fibres, pruritus and positive chronotropic action. These effects are basic to such conditions as urticaria, angio-oedema, asthma and anaphylactic shock.

For a long time, a clinical approach has induced a form of reasoning as follows: 'as there are urticarias caused by allergy to fish, then all fish-induced urticaria is due to allergy'. In fact the same symptom may be truly allergic, or simply a histamine reaction mediated by non-immunological mechanisms. We have suggested the term 'false food allergies' or 'pseudoallergic reactions to food' to characterize such eventualities (Moneret-Vautrin, 1983a). Others prefer either the terms, 'non-immuno-logical adverse reactions' or 'intolerance'.

Three types of mechanisms could be involved in false food allergy.

1. An abnormal intake of biogenic amines, such as histamine, tyramine and phenylethylamine (Moneret-Vautrin, 1991).
2. An abnormal release of chemical mediators from mast cells. The histamine mechanism is well identified, but other mediators derived from arachidonic acid may play a role. Skin mast cells seem to be susceptible to histamine-releasing agents. However, with regard to the location of histamine release in the gut, it is postulated that connective-type mast cells in the submucosa may be more prone to non-specific histamine release than mucosal mast cells (Moneret-Vautrin *et al.* 1984).
3. Interference by food or additives with the autonomic system (for review, see Moneret-Vautrin, 1986; Moneret-Vautrin and Maria, 1989).

PREVALENCE

Public perception of the detrimental effects of foodstuffs greatly exceeds the reality. Indeed, designing a questionnaire for epidemiological studies is obviously difficult, particularly when educated people are concerned. For example, the reported prevalence of adverse reactions to food was 33% in a group of teachers from London University (Bender and Matthews, 1981).

Food allergy may be present in 4–10% of children (Grogan, 1969; Buckley and Metcalfe, 1982; Rona and Chinn, 1987). False food allergy may be twice as frequent in children, who often have a high consumption

of histamine-releasing foods (e.g. strawberries and chocolate) and food colourings, preservatives and flavourings (May and Bock, 1978).

FOOD ALLERGENS: PROTEINS AND XENOBIOTICS

Food allergens are mainly proteins of average molecular mass, from 15 to 40 kDa; a single foodstuff can contain about 40 (Bleumink, 1970). One or two are major allergens, causing the appearance of specific IgE in 50% of subjects sensitized to the foodstuff (Baldo and Wrigley, 1978; Sachs *et al.* 1981; Langeland, 1983).

Modern techniques, such as polyacrylamide gel electrophoresis (PAGE), two-dimensional radioimmunoelectrophoresis and the immuno-blotting technique, allow antigenic fractions, including those promoting allergenicity, to be characterized in food extracts.

Antigenic determinants, or epitopes, are fragments of the amino acid sequence that combine specifically with antibodies. A protein molecule may contain many such epitopes. The determinant is said to be sequential if the nature and order only of the amino acids are necessary for its operation. It is then extremely resistant to any modification, like the allergen M of the cod (Elsayed and Apold, 1983).

Other determinants are conformational, in that the steric configuration of the polypeptide is essential for them to operate; they are thus easily denatured. These determinants are probably more common.

In the case of fruits and vegetables, allergens are easily denatured by phenol compounds and enzymes. Many antigenic determinants are ubiquitous, present as much in the various botanical families as in pollens (Hannuksela and Lahti, 1977; Bessot *et al.* 1984; Bernhisel-Broadbent, 1989). Some of them belong to the family of profilins, which are proteins that have been highly conserved during the evolutionary process (Valenta, 1992). Ripening increases the allergenicity considerably.

The allergenicity may depend on heating. It is assumed that allergens from plants such as banana, potato and apple are thermolabile, and allergens of animal origin are thermostable. Cooking, sterilization and storage under refrigeration do not diminish the allergenicity of fish or eggs (Tables 8.1 and 8.2). However, the albumins of various meats, egg and milk are thermolabile, whereas peanuts and tomato retain their allergenicity when heated.

Heating proteins with sugars may increase their allergenicity through an *N*-glycosidic linkage; the compounds so formed would be less easily hydrolysed by the processes of digestion (Bleumink, 1970). However, this assertion is controversial. In general, heat processing weakens the allergenicity of food proteins (Laughlan and Anderson, 1981), but it may enhance the allergenicity of others. During the denaturing of the protein,

Food allergy and intolerance in infancy

Table 8.1 Major allergenic proteins in foods from animal origin

Food allergen	Molecular mass (kDa)	Thermostability	Other characteristics
Milk			
β-Lactoglobulin	18	Yes	Products of digestion retain allergenic activity
α-Lactalbumin	16	No	
Caseins	20–24	Yes	
Serum albumin	69	No	Four Ig binding sites
Egg			
Ovomucoid	27–31	Yes	186 amino acids; sequence 69–130 thought to be allergenic
Ovotransferrin	82	No	
Ovalbumin	46	No	
Lysozyme	14	Yes	120 amino acids
Fish (cod)			
Allergen M (parvalbumin)	12	Yes	113 amino acids. Peptides 13–23, haptenic determinant; peptides 33–44, 65–74, 88–96, Ig binding sites
Shrimps			
SA-I	8.2		May be a fragment SA-II
SA-II	34		301 aminoacids

some reactive epitopes normally enclosed in the conformational structure may be unmasked. Küstner, who was a patient of Prausnitz, was allergic only to cooked fish (Prausnitz and Küstner, 1921).

Apart from the allergenicity, which is linked to the chemical structure, the sensitizing effect of food depends on the transfer of intact protein antigens to blood. Intraluminal and then intraenterocytic digestion operates on food proteins (Walker and Isselbacker, 1974). There are several possibilities of failure here. However, proteinase deficiency is never observed in food allergy. Neurovegetative disorders causing motor diarrhoea can induce maldigestion through insufficient substrate–enzyme contact time. However, their occurrence in patients with food allergy is not significant.

Table 8.2 Major allergenic proteins in food from fruit and vegetables

Food allergens	Molecular mass (kDa)	Thermostability	Other characteristics
Peanuts			
Arachin	180–330	Yes	22 allergens in crude extract
Conarachin I	140–295	Yes	10 in roasted peanuts
Conarachin A-reactive glycoprotein	–	Yes	
Tomatoes			
Glycoprotein	20–30	Yes	
Soyabeans			
Major allergen	20	Yes	
Kunitz inhibitor	–	–	
Wheat			
Globulins		Yes	Food allergy
Albumins		No	Baker's asthma
Starches		Yes	
Gliadin		Yes	Coeliac disease

The second barrier to the transfer of food allergens into the blood is the intestinal epithelium (Walker and Isselbacher, 1974). The physiological absorption of intact proteins is 1% in the healthy adult and a little more in the infant, but the premature infant is not at increased risk of food allergy. Absorption is higher in pathological conditions such as viral gastroenteritis, giardiasis and candidosis (Gruskay and Cooke, 1955; Heyman *et al.* 1987: Uhnoo *et al.* 1990). It is also increased by food sensitization, which induces local histamine release from mucosal mast cells. In this case, a vicious circle is set up: passage of the intact allergen, sensitization, hyperpermeability, easier passage, increased sensitization and so on (Dannaeus and Inganas, 1979).

For the clinician, it is obvious that the foods most incriminated are those most frequently consumed (flour and tomatoes in Italy, rice in Japan, fish in Scandinavia, peanuts in the USA). Peanuts seem to be extremely sensitizing since specific IgE are observed in very young infants who would be able to consume only small amounts of that particular allergen in the form of peanut butter (Table 8.3). We have drawn attention to the effects of masked peanut allergens present in milk formulas that contain peanut oil (Moneret-Vautrin *et al.* 1991). The predominance of allergens of animal origin is noteworthy, and is the reverse of the situation in the adult (Table 8.4).

Table 8.3 Food allergens[a] in 82 children aged from 5 months to 14 years

Food allergen	Percentage of cases	
1. Eggs	32.7%	}
2. Peanuts	18.6%	77% of cases
3. Fish	13.3%	
4. Milk	12.4%	
5. Beef	2.6%	}
6. Pork, shellfish	1.7%	12.8%
peas, cocoa beans		
hazel nuts, mustard		
12. Chicken, rabbit, garlic,	0.93%	}
soyabeans, sunflower,		10.2%
carrots, almonds,		
peaches, baker's yeast,		
wheat flour, azoic dyes		

[a]Allergy to the 21 food allergens was confirmed by prick tests, Rast and oral challenges. Allergy to azoic dyes was proved by oral challenges.

Table 8.4 Main food allergens[a] in 317 adults

Food allergen	Percentage	
1. Drupaceae[b]	16.6	}
2. Umbelliferae[c]	12	
3. Shellfish	11	64.5
4. Eggs	9.6	
5. Fish	9.3	
6. Milk	6	
7. Wheat	4	
8. Leguminosae[d]	3.3	
9. Mussels	3	
10. Potatoes	2.3	
11. Avocados	1.65	
12. Beef	1.65	
13. . . . and 41 other allergens		

[a]Allergy to the 53 allergens was diagnosed by positive prick test, Rast and oral challenges.
[b]Drupaceae: hazel nuts, apples, pears, plums, etc.
[c]Umbelliferae: celery, carrots, parsley, fennel, etc.
[d]Leguminosae: peas, haricot beans, soyabeans, etc.

Hypersensitivity to xenobiotics is a difficult challenge for the clinician. Those mainly involved are permitted additives such as colourings, preservatives and antioxidants, flavouring and texturizing agents. Thousands of these additives may be ingested, creating a new chemical microenvironment in the gut. IgE-dependent mechanisms involving additives have been

described, but in addition there are numerous pharmacological reactions that may be involved in adverse reactions to food. Azoic dyes, metabisulphites, benzoates and butylhydroxytoluene are particularly involved (Michaelsson and Juhlin, 1973; Freedman, 1977; Moneret-Vautrin and Aubert, 1978; Wüthrich, 1983; Pollock, 1991). We stress the frequency of delayed type of sensitization to vanilla or vanillin in young children with atopic dermatitis (Table 8.5).

CLINICAL CHARACTERISTICS OF FOOD ALLERGY

Atopy is almost always to be found in children with food allergy. We conducted a survey in 35 children with food allergy and found that in 91% of cases there was a previous history of atopic dermatitis, either alone or associated with asthma. Upon diagnosis of food allergy, 81% of the children had atopic dermatitis, 37% had a respiratory allergy and 85.3% of epidermal prick tests were positive with inhalants (Table 8.6).

Food allergy is incriminated in atopic dermatitis, respiratory allergy, urticaria, recurring angio-oedema, anaphylactic shock and recurring idiopathic anaphylaxis, nephrotic syndrome, recurring serous otitis and other conditions (Moneret-Vautrin and André, 1983; Sampson *et al.* 1989).

Table 8.5 Double blind oral provocation tests in 11 children with atopic dermatitis

No.	Sex	Age	Placebo	Peru balsam	Vanilla	Vanillin
1.	F	3.5 years	2 : −	−		
2.	F	2.5 years	1 : −	+		
3.	M	13 months	1 : −	+		
4.	F	2.5 years	1 : −	++		
5.	M	10 months	1 : −	+		
7.	F	31.5 months	2 : −		−	+
8.	F	4 years	4 : −		−	−
9.	M	12 months	1 : −		++(as)[a]	++
10.	F	21.5 months	1 : −	+	[b]	+
11.	M	10 months	4 : 2− : 2+−		+	+
12.	M	5 years	1 : −		−	+

[a]Associated with vanillin.
[b]Test not performed.
−, Negative; +, exacerbation of eczema: ++, strongly positive.

Table 8.6 Detection of atopy in 34 children with food allergy from 8 months to 12 years

Clinical diseases	Percentage	Positive prick tests	Percentage
Atopic dermatitis alone	55.8	House dust mites	55
Asthma and rhinitis	8.8	Pollens	55
Atopic dermatitis and asthma	26.4	Animal epithelia	43
Total with clinical disease	91.0	Moulds	3
No clinical disease	9.0	Total positive to prick tests	85.3
		No reaction to prick tests	14.7

Atopic dermatitis

Atopic dermatitis is a multifaceted disorder, affecting 5–6% of children. The triggering role of food allergy has long been proposed because of the frequency of specific IgE and the aggravation caused by certain foodstuffs (Pike and Atherton, 1987). Formal confirmation rests on challenges and on the curing of inflammation by an elimination diet (Sampson and McCaskill, 1985). It seems reasonable to postulate that 35% of atopic dermatitis cases are largely due to food allergy (Burks *et al.* 1988). Indeed, the skin of an atopic dermatitis patient has a high tendency towards histamine release from the sensitized mast cells when the antigen arrives through the bloodstream. An eosinophilic cellular infiltration is also created, with deposits of MBP (major basic protein). Sensitized T-lymphocytes release a cytokine, histamine-releasing factor, which makes the basophils abnormally fragile to histamine release (Sampson *et al.* 1989). These lymphocytes can be actived by Langerhans cells, which are themselves activated if food allergens bind with specific IgE on their surface (Buckley, 1989; Bruijnzeel-Koomen *et al.* 1989). Polysensitization to food is common: milk, eggs and peanuts are the main foods involved. Reactions to additives are also frequent, and flavourings need to be considered.

Asthma

Asthma would seem to be related to a food allergy in 8% of cases (Moneret-Vautrin, 1987a). The most frequent condition is an allergy to fruits and vegetables in subjects sensitized to birch pollens. This explains why asthma related to food allergy is much more common in England and northern France than in countries like Spain. The involvement of multiple additives needs to be systematically studied. Respiratory-type intolerance to metabisulphite, sodium benzoate, tartrazine and other colouring products would seem to affect 11% of asthmatics (Freedman, 1977).

Rhinitis

In 20% of rhinitis cases, there is a coexisting food allergy. However, a causal link has been established in fewer than 4% of patients. As in the case of asthma, cross-reactivity amongst fruits, vegetables and pollens explains the presence of IgE specific to these foodstuffs without there being any clinical symptoms (Mouton and Moneret-Vautrin, 1988). In patients with pollinosis and cross-allergy to foods, the oral syndrome, which was first described by Lessof, is much more frequent than nasal symptoms.

Urticaria and oedema

Chronic urticaria and Quinke's oedema (angio-oedema) are the most common manifestations of food allergy, occurring in more than 70% of patients. Conversely, food allergy is involved in no more than 5% of chronic urticaria cases. Exceptional cases of urticaria with vasculitis and associated purpura, or of purpura alone, have been linked to such foods as blackberries, tartrazine and butyl hydroxytoluene (BHT). Exertion urticaria can be the prodrome of exertion anaphylaxis. Chronic urticaria is often non-immunological, but pseudoallergic reactions to food are quite common.

The localization of angio-oedema on the lips, uvula, or pharynx and larynx, as well as dysphagia at the level of the superior oesophagus, are strongly suggestive of an allergy to fruits or vegetables in a patient sensitized to pollens. Indeed, this corresponds to maximum tissue sensitization to inhaled pollens of the aero-digestive junction, where fruit and vegetable antigens react with anti-pollen specific IgE. However, the infant often presents a laryngeal oedema as a manifestation of food allergy, even to allergens of animal origin.

Anaphylactic shock

Anaphylactic shock is linked to food allergy in 6% of cases. The signs occur within minutes of ingesting the foodstuff. Itching of the lips and palate and oedema of the buccal mucosa sometimes constitute its prodrome. Then urticaria and angio-oedema become generalized, and a bronchospasm occurs with tachycardia and collapse followed by epigastralgia, stomach pains and diarrhoea. The speed with which the shock sets in often leads the family to correctly suspect the foodstuff concerned, unless the food allergen is hidden in the food. This raises the issue of informative labelling. If such is not the case and no diagnosis is reached, the condition may recur (idiopathic recurring anaphylaxis). Shock is rare in children. In infants, it would seem to represent no more than 5% of

cases of intolerance to cows' milk proteins. Oral challenge after 2 weeks elimination of milk could be a special risk.

Nephrotic syndrome

The role of food allergy in nephrotic syndrome with corticosensitive, minimal glomerular lesions seems to be established (Sandberg, 1977). The incidence of atopic diseases in children with nephrotic syndrome has been estimated as 25–33%, and food allergy could account for 2.6–3.8% of cases (Lin *et al.* 1990). No local deposit of IgE or semi-delayed inflammatory reaction has been demonstrated, and it is suggested that the condition may be mediated by non-IgE mechanisms.

Many other clinical conditions have been attributed to a food allergy: serous otitis, eosinophilic gastroenteritis, infantile colic, irritable colon syndrome, rheumatoid purpura, membranoproliferative glomerulonephritis, ocular allergies, Heiner's syndrome, sudden infant death and so on (Heiner *et al.* 1962; Moneret-Vautrin, 1983b; Sampson, 1989a; Barau and Dupont, 1990).

The tension–fatigue syndrome described by Randolph and then by Speer, and psychomotor agitation (Feinberg's syndrome of the hyperactive child), have in no way been linked to an immunologically defined food allergy. Rare cases might nevertheless be related to intolerance to additives via unidentified mechanisms (Pollock, 1991). Interference of certain chemical products with different kinds of neurotransmission has been postulated and, according to some experimental studies, is plausible.

Development of childhood food allergy

The normal development of food allergy in the child depends on many factors. Except for the case of cows' milk protein intolerance, which often disappears at about 2 years, food allergy is long-lasting. After 5 years a cure is obtained in only 31–45% of cases (Bock, 1982, 1986, 1989; Sampson and Scanlon, 1989; Businco *et al.* 1989). Subjects who have not been cured present either persisting clinical symptoms, or biological indicators of hypersensitivity associated with a clinical state of partial tolerance (Bock and Atkins, 1990). The acquisition of this tolerance can be observed clinically while histamine release from basophils and digestive mast cells is still provoked by the presence of the allergen. This effect disappears, but specific IgE may persist as long as 10 years after the allergy. Finally, the IgE antibodies disappear (Dannaeus and Inganas, 1981; Moneret-Vautrin, 1983b; Moneret-Vautrin and André, 1983).

This course of events depends on the nature of the allergens: milk, soya, citrus fruits and eggs would seem to be more rapidly tolerated than peanuts, fish or crustacea (Dannaeus and Inganas, 1979, Bock, 1982).

The time scale is shorter in cases of monosensitization than in cases of polysensitization. Generally, the earlier in life food allergy appears, the earlier it is cured (Bock, 1982, 1986; Businco *et al.* 1989). The intensity of the sensitization influences how long the allergy persists: the specific IgE content is seven times lower in children who eventually become tolerant than in those who continue to present with allergy. Similarly, the non-acquisition of specific IgG could characterize the persistence of allergy (Dannaeus and Inganas, 1981). When the food allergy causes atopic dermatitis, it may also be observed that children presenting typical symptoms will be cured far more often than those with atypical lesions (Businco *et al.* 1989).

PSEUDOALLERGIC REACTIONS TO FOOD IN CHILDREN

Not only children with atopic dermatitis, but also those with allergic asthma or hay fever are at risk of pseudoallergic reactions to food. In fact, the abnormal tendency of atopic patients to release histamine is well known, as basophils exhibit an appreciable spontaneous histamine release. Many foodstuffs may possess a histamine-releasing effect, including egg ovomucoid (all the more so since it is raw), crustaceans, strawberries, chocolate, tomatoes, pineapple and pawpaw. If the child is greedy, the ingestion of such food relative to body weight may be excessive.

As eczematous skin is rich in mast cells, histamine will be released in greater quantities, and the lesions will be worsened by scratching. Once the child is cured of dermatitis, the same food is tolerated, instead of eliciting reactions as would be the case with true allergy. Other clinical symptoms are urticaria and angio-oedema.

The growing child becomes less sensitive to histamine release. After 8–10 years of age, pseudoallergic reactions become less common, unless the diet is extremely unbalanced.

Other foods are rich in histamine (fermented food), tyramine (chocolate) or serotonin (banana). Either by direct action or by their histamine-releasing action, these biogenic amines can induce pseudoallergic reactions.

Finally, intolerance to additives plays an increasing role in pseudoallergic reactions: azo dyes, preservatives (benzoic acid, butyl hydroxytoluene, antioxidants, metabisulphites) and are only a few examples of those identified among xenobiotics. The extended use of flavourings has to be considered insofar as some (vanilla and synthetic vanillin) have already been implicated. A noxious role for vegetable gums is now suspected.

DIAGNOSIS

The diagnostic procedure involves several stages and efficient implement-ation demands great care (Fig. 8.1). A dietary history is elicited by question-ing, and completed by a study of food intake. The interview aims to detect possible atopy in the family and atopic symptoms in the child. The daily consumption of certain foodstuffs or, in contrast, the disgust elicited by cer-tain foodstuffs, can lead one to suspect food allergy and to seek a chronolog-ical relation between the intake of a particular foodstuff and the appearance of symptoms. Careful observations of the parents are worth taking into ac-count. However, the overall efficiency of the questioning is fairly low.

Dietary history

For this reason, the search for an alimentary cause begins with the study of the patient's diet over a period of a week. A child's parents note down all the food and liquid consumed, together with the quantities.

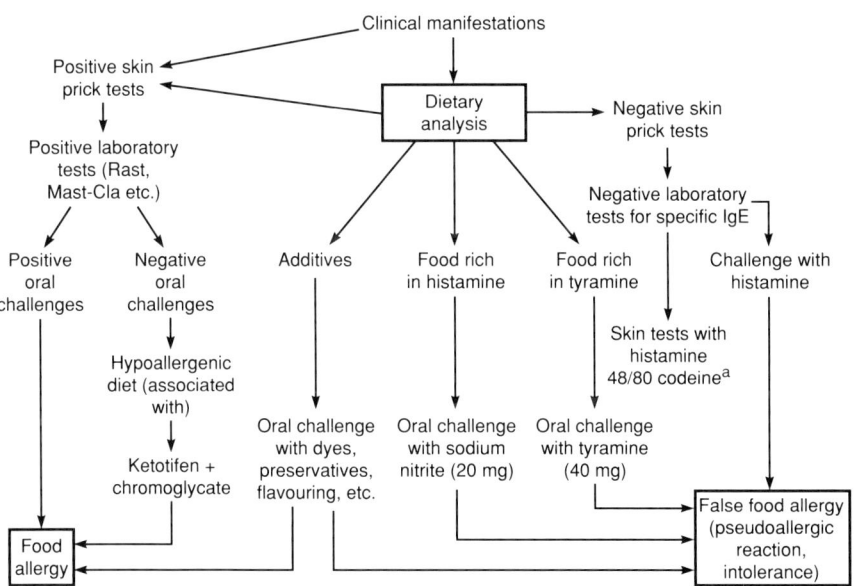

[a]Evaluation of abnormal histamine release, and abnormal response to histamine

[b]Not done in children (see Bock, 1982)

Figure 8.1 Diagnosis of food allergy and pseudoallergic reactions (intolerance) to foods. Even if SPT are negative, a clinical suspicion should lead to laboratory tests for IgE antibodies. If the latter are negative, a food allergy may be discarded, cow milk allergy being excluded.

The complete composition of all manufactured foods must be noted in order to detect excessive consumption of additives, and possible 'hidden' food allergens. We emphasize that taking a dietary history by questionnaire is the indispensable preliminary to any allergy investigation. Just as each individual's dressing habits differ from those of his or her neighbours, so do his or her eating habits. Although it is true that about 30 common food allergens account for most allergies, it is also true that in each case rarer allergens suggested by the dietary history must be considered.

Tests for IgE-dependent allergy

The demonstration of sensitization begins with epidermal prick tests. Superficial, painless and harmless, these tests are both sensitive and specific, and can be used on babies only a few months of age. They are carried out using about 40 commercial allergenic extracts or the native foodstuff ground into a little physiological saline. The diameter of the wheal is compared with a negative control with saline and a positive control with codeine. Criteria of positivity have been established (Bock *et al.* 1978). Their negative predictive accuracy is over 95%.

These tests are useful for selecting the foodstuffs for which to search for specific IgE using the radioallergosorbent test (Rast). The specificity and sensitivity of tests for specific IgE to food are high with radioisotopic techniques (Rast Phadebas) but lower with immunoenzymic techniques. Thus there is an increased risk of a false negative test if the latter tests are used (Moneret-Vautrin *et al.* 1990a). However, the liquid phase technique, in which the allergen is bound to a soluble matrix, provides a real improvement (Moneret-Vautrin *et al.* 1993).

Other available tests include the Mast-Cla multi-detection test, which yields information on 36 food allergens (Moneret-Vautrin *et al.* 1990b) and the basophil histamine-release assay, which has to be performed carefully, as the high spontaneous histamine release makes the interpretation difficult in some cases (Sampson *et al.* 1989). A good correlation with Rast and skin tests and even intestinal mast cell histamine release has been demonstrated (Nolte *et al.* 1989).

Clinical tests

The involvement of specific IgE in clinical symptoms relies on carefully scrutinized challenge tests. Double-blind challenges represent the gold standard of food allergy diagnosis. However, with young children, single-blind or open oral challenges are sufficient.

It is advisable to carry out the tests in a medical setting after 2 weeks elimination of the foodstuff in cases of chronic diseases such as atopic

dermatitis. Any antihistamine medication must be suspended long enough to allow histamine reactivity of the skin to be restored. The challenge is carried out on a fasting patient, either with a lyophilized extract or with ground or mashed foodstuff mixed with a non-allergizing foodstuff to disguise it (apple sauce, apple juice or mashed potatoes). In general, the first dose of 250 mg is doubled every 30 minutes up to 10 g (Sampson, 1989b).

In case of anaphylaxis we recommend a labial challenge before the oral one by putting a drop of the extract in solution (or of the native foodstuff) on the lower lip. A positive reaction is characterized by a sometimes extensive oedema of the lip, occurring in under 15 minutes (Fig. 8.2). If there is no reaction, we give 5–30 g orally, depending on the symptoms and age of the child.

The oral challenge can be coupled with an intestinal permeability test, when the changes observed provide substantial additional supporting evidence for interpreting challenge tests as positive (Dupont *et al.* 1989).

The period of observation necessary is up to 2 hours for IgE-mediated reactions, up to 6 hours for digestive reactions and up to 48–72 hours for atopic dermatitis. In the last case, the additives incriminated in the alimentary investigation can be double-blind tested at home. When an attack of eczema follows an oral challenge, the other tests are postponed and a test treatment with disodium chromoglycate and ketotifen is instituted. A positive result can be considered as pointing to food allergy.

Oral challenges, if carried out following a strict protocol, give accurate

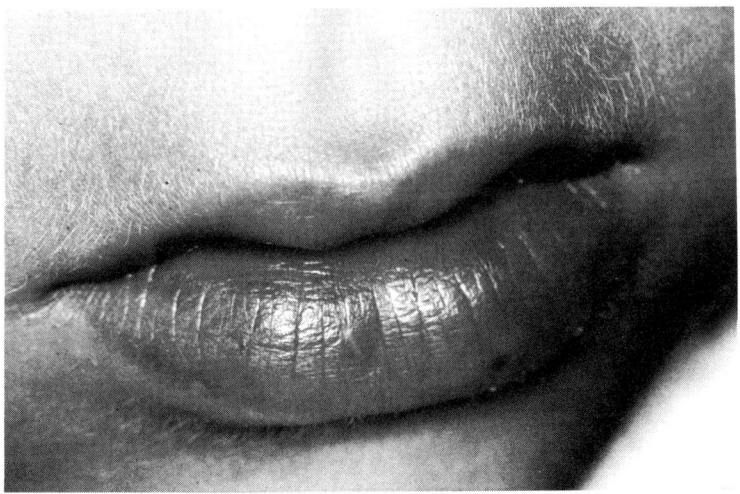

Figure 8.2 Labial food challenge in a child sensitized to egg. Extensive oedema of the lower lip can be seen 15 minutes after a drop of raw egg white is place on the lip.

results for food allergies in 94.5% of cases. The rate of false negative tests would seem to be 4.6% and that of false positive tests 0.9% (Sampson, 1989b; Bock and Atkins, 1990). However, not all types of food allergy give such good results. Diagnosing food allergy remains difficult in cases of asthma or nephrotic syndrome. The oral challenge may be impossible to interpret owing to lack of objective clinical symptoms. A negative oral challenge under basal conditions cannot completely rule out the possibility of food allergy. Even positive responses may give rise to doubt: do they show that there is food allergy or subclinical manifestations of sensitization? In such cases, it might be postulated that factors such as exertion and allergenic stimulation by pollen in the appropriate season may produce symptoms.

In nephropathies with minimal glomerular lesions, it is necessary to impose a strict daily study, spread over several days, of renal functions (24-hour proteinuria, weight and so on) after a challenge, while the child is kept on a strict diet and fed parenterally with amino acids (Lagrue and Laurent, 1982).

Other tests and measurements have been suggested: plasma histamine, serum tryptase, endoscopy and biopsy of digestive mucosa after instillation of allergen extract, looking for Charcot–Leyden crystals and quantifying IgE in faeces, and measuring urinary methylhistamine. However, these tests are of only general value. The assessment of the basal intestinal permeability could be interesting. Indeed, the existence of a hyperpermeability is a good prognostic factor for the efficiency of drugs such as disodium chromoglycate or anti-H_1.

When there is a cause-and-effect relationship between food and symptoms, and all investigations have failed to establish a food allergy, a moderately restrictive hypoallergenic diet may be given for 6 weeks. A successful result justifies repeat investigations. If no improvement is observed, food allergy is unlikely. Even if a diagnosis of food allergy can be discarded, i.e. an immunological mechanism can be ruled out, it is still necessary to search for pseudoallergic reactions (Fig. 8.1).

TREATMENT

There are six general rules.

1. First of all, if the food allergy is severe, it is important to explain to the parents, teachers and child how to eliminate the foodstuff completely. Some suggest giving the child a bracelet or necklace to wear with the name of the foodstuff on it. However, complete elimination is difficult, and it must be remembered that 1 mg is enough to trigger a shock. Indeed, in 32 subjects allergic to peanuts, 16 had a reaction after

accidental ingestion (Bock, 1989). In the case of anaphylaxis, the child must be given a first-aid bag with injectable adrenalin and oral corticosteroids (Committee report of the AAAI, 1991).

2. In order to minimize the consequences of accidental ingestion, the mucosa must be protected daily with disodium chromoglycate, of which an average dose of 300 mg must be taken three times a day, 45 minutes before meals (Businco & Cantani, 1990). Combination with antihistamine drugs such as ketotifen, loratadine, cetirizine or oxatomide is advisable. However, such treatment is only partly successful. Under no circumstances does pharmacological treatment alone succeed in eliminating risk completely.

3. All causes of irritation and hyperpermeability of the intestinal mucosa must be avoided: spices, acetylsalicylic acid and, to a lesser extent, non-steroid anti-inflammatory drugs. Giardiasis or the presence of large quantities of intestinal yeasts must be eradicated.

4. In case of monosensitization, the key to preventing further accidents is complete elimination. If the child is allergic to cows' milk, it is illogical to use foods containing sensitizing proteins such as soya or goats' milk as substitutes. So-called hypoallergenic milks based on whey hydrolysates are potentially reactogenic for the sensitized child. Casein hydrolysates supplying peptides of <3500 Da should be used. In allergy to egg, one should be suspicious of foodstuffs developed for athletes and body-builders, which are powders made from egg, soya or milk proteins, of medicines containing lysozyme, and of certain antiviral vaccines (German measles, measles, mumps and amaril fever). In allergy to fish, surimi should be avoided. Although not obvious, it can be present in certain culinary preparations. Allergy to peanuts is a major problem in children: it is the most common allergy in the USA, and second in France. Giving very young children biscuits that may contain peanut butter or milk formulas containing peanut oil represents a serious risk today. Monosensitizations to other fruits and vegetables are less common in children, and cooking lessens their allergenicity.

5. In cases of polysensitization, challenge tests are of paramount importance: they must be carried out to distinguish between symptomatic allergies and latent sensitizations. Indeed, the latter are much more common, and positive prick tests might be misinterpreted as food allergies. Therefore, challenge tests are invaluable in restricting the number of foods to be eliminated, thus reducing the risk of nutritional deficiencies.

6. When the diet is unbalanced, the aim is no longer one of eradication but of restriction, either of starchy foods, or of foods rich in tyramine, histamine, histamine-releasing foods, or additives, according to

circumstances. It must be borne in mind that an allergy is often associated with a pseudoallergy, and that both must be taken into account when prescribing a diet to bring about a distinct improvement (Ventura *et al.* 1989). While taking account of these requirements, one must both ensure safety and avoid unjustified diets that may induce deficiencies. In a study by Weber on 73 children with atopic dermatitis, 71% were on diets with no scientific basis, some of which were sensitizing, and 6% were on diets that were dangerous in terms of nutritional balance. One should aim for rational elimination diets to achieve parental confidence and consequently improved compliance (Hathaway and Warner, 1983).

The study of food allergy in children shows that it is a long-term affair. The recent study by Sampson and Scanlon (1989) reported spontaneous recovery after 1 year in only 26% of cases. After 2 or even 3 years, the percentage was only a little higher. This is why, in cases of severe food allergy in which elimination is difficult, we now suggest hyposensitization by subcutaneous injection subsequently boosted by progressive oral habituation. This method gives good results (Moneret-Vautrin, 1987b). Others use the oral pathway alone (Wüthrich and Hofer, 1986).

PREVENTION OF SENSITIZATION TO FOOD ALLERGENS

The fetus can be sensitized *in utero*. Moreover, the incidence of allergy to milk and even to other food proteins is higher in atopic families. It was consequently suggested that eggs, fish, peanut and milk be avoided during the last 3 months of pregnancy, the mother also taking disodium chromoglycate. However, no positive result was achieved (Fälth-Magnusson *et al.* 1987).

Similarly, tests involving prolonged exclusive breast feeding of atopic babies by mothers on a hypoallergenic diet have yielded no conclusive evidence. Chandra *et al.* (1989) concluded that an appropriate diet during pregnancy, and exclusive breast feeding are very beneficial. Hattevig *et al.* (1984) was less categorical, since they observed a lower frequency of atopic dermatitis in the early months followed by a poorer outcome at 9 months. Zeiger *et al.* (1989) observed a reduced incidence of food allergies at age 12 months, but no significant difference at 24 months in the incidence of rhinitis and asthma. Numerous publications are devoted to the results of hypoallergenic diets both for mothers during pregnancy and breast feeding, and for infants. However, approximately equal numbers in each of these three categories conclude that the approach is, and is not, beneficial.

For the time being it can be concluded that the ideas are intellectually

exciting, but so far unproved by experience. We suggest that starting the diet for the pregnant woman in the last months of pregnancy might be too late, owing to the possibilities of immune response in the younger fetus. On the other hand, the prevention of allergic diseases should not be restricted to avoidance of food allergens, but should simultaneously include great care about pollutants such as tobacco and inhalants.

CONCLUSIONS

Eating habits have changed more in the last 40 years than from prehistoric times up to the Second World War. Some of these changes may contribute towards a microenvironment damaging to the digestive tract in the same way as airborne allergens and atmospheric pollution constitute a damaging environment for the respiratory tract. Food allergy and pseudoallergic reactions (or intolerance) are the price we have to pay for allowing this environmental hazard to exist. Any agroalimentary technology that modifies food proteins or introduces xenobiotics creates new risks and we can safely predict the widespread extension of this pathology. Consequently, the concept of hypoallergenicity of processed nutriments, although still in its early theoretical stages, should open up interesting possibilities for research and for applications to human nutrition (Moneret-Vautrin, 1988).

REFERENCES

Baldo, B.A. and Wrigley, C.W. (1978) IgE antibodies to wheat flour components; studies with sera from subjects with baker's asthma or coeliac condition. *Clinical Allergy*, 8, 109–124.

Barau, E. and Dupont, C. (1990) Modifications of intestinal permeability during food provocation procedures in pediatric irritable bowel syndrome. *Journal of Pediatric Gastroenterology and Nutrition*, 11, 72–77.

Bender, A.E. and Matthews, D.R. (1981) Adverse reactions to food. *British Journal of Nutrition*, 46, 403–407.

Bernhisel-Broadbent, J. (1989) Cross-allergenicity in the legume botanical family in children with food hypersensitivity. *Journal of Allergy and Clinical Immunology*, 83, 435–440.

Bessot, J.C., Dietemann-Molard, A., Braun, P.A. and Pauli, G. (1984) [The associations of pollinosis with Betulaceae and food allergy with apples and other plants.] *Revue Française Allergologie*, 24, 29–33.

Bleumink, E. (1970) Food allergy: the chemical nature of the substances eliciting symptoms. *World Review of Nutrition and Dietetics*, 12, 505–507.

Bock, S.A. (1982) The natural history of food sensitivity. *Journal of Allergy and Clinical Immunology*, 69, 173–177.

Bock, S.A. (1986) The natural history of adverse reactions to food. *New England and Regional Allergy Proceedings*, 7, 504–510.

Bock, S.A. (1989) The natural history of peanut allergy. *Journal of Allergy and Clinical Immunology*, 83, 900–904.

Bock, S.A. and Atkins, F.M. (1990) Patterns of food hypersensitivity during sixteen years of double-blind placebo-controlled food challenges. *Journal of Pediatrics*, 117, 561–567.

Bock, S.A., Buckley, J., Holst, A. and May, C.D. (1978) Proper use of skin tests with food extracts in diagnosis of food hypersensitivity. *Clinical Allergy*, 8, 559–564.

Bruijnzeel-Koomen, C., Bieber, T., Mudde, G. and Bruijnzeel, P. (1989) New aspects in the pathogenesis of atopic dermatitis: the role of epidermal Langerhans cells. *Allergologie*, 12, 150–154.

Buckley, R.J. (1989) IgE and the pathogenesis of atopic eczema. In *Progress in Allergy and Clinical Immunology*, pp. 336–339 (eds W.J. Pichler, B.M. Stadler, C.A. Dahinden, A.R. Pecoud, P. Frei, C.H. Schneider and A.L. de Weck). Bern: Hogrefe & Huber.

Buckley, R.H. and Metcalfe, D. (1982) Food allergy. *Journal of the American Medical Association*, 248, 26–27.

Burks, A.W., Mallort, S.B., Williams L.W. and Shirrell, M.A. (1988) Atopic dermatitis: clinical relevance of food hypersensitivity reactions. *Journal of Pediatrics*, 113, 447–451.

Businco, L. and Cantani, A. (1990) Food allergy in children: diagnosis and treatment with sodium chromoglycate. *Allergologie Immunopathologie*, 18, 339–348.

Businco, L., Ziruolo, M.G., Ferrara, M. *et al.* (1989) Natural history of atopic dermatitis in childhood: an updated review and personal experience of a five-year follow-up. *Allergy*, 44, (Suppl. 9), 70–78.

Chandra, R.K., Puri, S. and Hamed, A. (1989) Influence of maternal diet during lactation and use of formula feeds on development of atopic eczema in high risk infants. *British Medical Journal*, 299, 228–230.

Committee Report from the Adverse Reactions to Food Committee of the American Academy of Allergy and Immunology (1991) The treatment in school of children who have food allergies. *Journal of Allergy and Clinical Immunology*, 87, 749–751.

Dannaeus, A. and Inganas, M. (1979) Intestinal uptake of ovalbumin in malabsorption and food allergy in relation to serum IgG antibody and orally administrated sodium chromoglycate. *Clinical Allergy*, 9, 263–270.

Dannaeus, A. and Inganas, M. (1981) A follow-up study of children with food allergy: clinical course in relation to serum IgE and IgG antibody levels to milk egg and fish. *Clinical Allergy*, 11, 533–539.

Dupont, C., Barau, E., Molkhou, P. *et al.* (1989) Food-induced alteration of intestinal permeability in children with cow's milk sensitive enteropathy and atopic dermatitis. *Journal of Pediatric Gastroenterology and Nutrition*, 8, 459–465.

Elsayed, S. and Apold J. (1983) Immunochemical analysis of cod fish allergen M: locations of the immunoglobulin binding sites as demonstrated by the native and synthetic peptides. *Allergy*, 38, 449–459.

Fälth-Magnusson, K., Oman, H. and Kjellman, N.I.M. (1987) Maternal abstention from cow milk and egg in allergy risk pregnancies: effect on antibody production in the mother and the newborn. *Allergy*, 42, 64–73.

Freedman, B.J. (1977) Asthma induced by sulphur dioxide, benzoate and tartrazine contained in orange drinks. *Clinical Allergy*, 7, 407–415.

Grogan, F.T. (1969) Food allergy in children after infancy. *Pediatric Clinics of North America*, 16, 217–225.

Gruskay, F.L. and Cooke, R.E. (1955) The gastrointestinal absorption of unaltered protein in normal infants and in infants recovering from diarrhea. *Pediatrics*, 16, 763–769.

Hannuksela, M. and Lahti, A. (1977) Immediate reactions to fruits and vegetables. *Contact Dermatitis*, **3**, 79–87.

Hathaway, M.J. and Warner, J.O. (1983) Compliance problems in the dietary management of eczema. *Archives of Diseases in Childhood*, **58**, 463–464.

Hattevig, G., Kjellman, B., Johansson, S.G.O. and Bjorksten, B. (1984) Clinical symptoms and IgE responses to common food proteins in atopic and healthy children. *Clinical Allergy*, **14**, 551.

Hattevig, G., Kjellman, B. and Bjorksten, B. (1987) Clinical symptoms and IgE responses to common food proteins and inhalants: the first seven years of life. *Clinical Allergy*, **17**, 571–578.

Heiner, D.C., Sears, J.W. *et al.* (1962) Multiple precipitins to cow's milk in chronic respiratory disease. *American Journal of Diseases of Children*, **103**, 634–654.

Heyman, M., Corthier, G., Petit, A. *et al.* (1987) Intestinal absorption of macromolecules during viral enteritis: an experimental study on rotavirus-infected conventional and germ-free mice. *Pediatric Research*, **22**, 72–78.

Lagrue, G. and Laurent, J. (1982) [Role of allergy in lipid-associated nephritis.] *La Nouvelle Presse Medicale*, **11**, 1465–1466.

Langeland, T. (1983) A clinical and immunological study of allergy to hen's egg white related to clinical and immunological parameters in egg-allergic patients. *Allergy*, **38**, 493–500.

Laughlan, P.M. and Anderson, K.J. (1981) Effect of heat on the anaphylactic sensitizing capacity of cow's milk, goat's milk and various infant formulae fed to guinea-pigs. *Archives of Diseases in Childhood*, **56**, 165–171.

Lin, C.Y., Lee, B.H., Lin, C.C. and Chen, W.P. (1990) A study of the relationship between childhood nephrotic syndrome and allergic diseases. *Chest*, **97**, 1408–1411.

Matsumura, T. and Kuroume, T. (1975) Egg sensitivity and eczematous manifestations in breast-fed newborns with particular reference to intra-uterine sensitization. *Annals of Allergy*, **35**, 221–229.

May, C.D. and Bock, S.A. (1978) Adverse reactions to food due to hypersensivity. In *Allergy, Principles and Practice*, pp. 1159–1171 (eds E. Middleton, C.E. Reed and E.F. Ellis). St Louis, MO: Mosby.

Michaelsson, G. and Juhlin, L. (1973) Urticaria induced by preservatives and dye additives in food and drugs. *British Journal of Dermatology*, **88**, 525–538.

Moneret-Vautrin, D.A. (1983a) False food allergies: non-specific reactions to foodstuffs. In *Clinical Reactions to Food*, pp. 135–153 (ed. M.H. Lessof). New York: Wiley.

Moneret-Vautrin, D.A. (1983b) Hypersensitivity to milk in adults: present aspects. In *Milk Intolerance and Rejection*, pp. 138–141 (ed. J. Delmont). Basel: Karger.

Moneret-Vautrin, D.A. (1986) Food antigens and additives. *Journal of Allergy and Clinical Immunology*, **78**, 1039–1046.

Moneret-Vautrin, D.A. (1987a) Food-related asthma. In *Highlights in Asthmology*, pp. 359–363. Berlin: Springer-Verlag.

Moneret-Vautrin, D.A. (1987b) [Immunotherapy and food allergy.] In *Jornada Internacional de Alergia Alimentaria*, pp. 97–104 (ed. J. Botey). (Proceedings of workshop, Barcelona).

Moneret-Vautrin, D.A. (1988) [Prevention of food allergy: is it possible?] *Revue Français Allergologie*, **28**, 287–295.

Moneret-Vautrin, D.A. (1991) Biogenic amines. In *Food Allergy and Food Intolerance*, pp. 61–71 (eds J.C. Somogyi, H.R. Müller and Th. Ockhuissen). Basel: Karger.

Moneret-Vautrin, D.A. and André, Cl. (1983) [Immunopathology of food allergy and false food allergy.] Paris: Masson.

Moneret-Vautrin, D.A. and Aubert B. (1978) [Risk of sensitization to food and drug colours.] Paris: Masson.

Moneret-Vautrin, D.A. and Maria, Y. (1989) Pseudo-allergic reactions to food. In *Food Allergy in Infancy and Childhood*, pp. 53–60 (eds H.K. Harms and U. Wahn). Berlin: Springer-Verlag.

Moneret-Vautrin, D.A., de Korwin, J.D., Tisserant, J. *et al.* (1984) Ultrastructural study of the mast cells of the human duodenal mucosa. *Clinical Allergy*, **14**, 471–481.

Moneret-Vautrin, D.A., Guéant, J.L., Abdel-Ghani, A., *et al.* (1990a). Comparative evaluation between two immunoenzymatic techniques (Fast and Phadezym) and the Phadebas Rast in food allergy. *Allergy*, **45**, 104–108.

Moneret-Vautrin, D.A., Kanny, G., Gerard, H. *et al.* (1990b) [Determination of specific IgE in food allergy by MAST-CLA: correlation with skin tests and RAST.] *Revue Français Allergologie*, **30**, 225–231.

Moneret-Vautrin, D.A., Hatahet, R., Kanny, G. and Ait Djafer, Z. (1991) Allergenic peanut oil in milk formulas. *Lancet*, **338**, 1149.

Moneret-Vautrin, D.A., Halpern, G.M., Brignon, J.J. *et al.* (1993) Food specific IgE antibodies: a comparative study of AlaSTAT and Pharmacia RAST Phadebas CAP systems in 49 patients with food allergies. *Annals of Allergy*, **71**, 107–114.

Mouton, C. and Moneret-Vautrin, D.A. (1988) Frequency of food allergy in chronic rhinitis, both allergic and non-allergic: study of 135 cases by skin tests, TDBH and challenge tests. *Médecine et Hygiène*, **46**, 1665–1669.

Nolte, H., Schiotz, P.O., Kruse, A. and Skov S. (1989) Comparison of intestinal mast cell and basophil histamine release in children with food allergic reactions. *Allergy*, **44**, 554–565.

Pike, M. and Atherton, D.J. (1987) Atopic eczema. In *Food Allergy*, pp. 583–601 (eds J. Brostoff and S. J. Challacombe). London: Ballière & Tindal.

Pollock, I. (1991) Hyperactivity and food additives. In *Food Allergy and Food Intolerance*, pp. 81–89 (eds J. C. Somogyi, H. R. Müller and Th. Ockhuisen). Basel: Karger.

Prausnitz, O.C. and Küstner, H. (1921) [Studies on hypersensitivity.] *Zentralblatt für Bakteriologie, Parasitenkunde Infektionskrankheiten und Hygiene*, **86**, 160–161.

Rona, R.J. and Chinn, S. (1987) Parent's perceptions of food intolerance in primary school children. *British Medical Journal*, **294**, 863–866.

Sachs, M.I., Jones, R.T. and Yunginger, J.W. (1981) Isolation and partial characterization of a major peanut allergen. *Journal of Allergy and Clinical Immunology*, **67**, 27–34.

Sampson, H.A. (1989a) Infantile colic and food allergy: fact or fiction? *Journal of Pediatrics*, **115**, 583–584.

Sampson, H.A. (1989b) Food allergy. *Journal of Allergy and Clinical Immunology*, **84**, 1062–1067.

Sampson, H.A. and McCaskill, C.C. (1985) Food hypersensitivity and atopic dermatitis: evaluation of 113 patients. *Journal of Pediatrics*, **107**, 669–675

Sampson, H.A. and Scanlon, S.M. (1989) Natural history of food hypersensitivity in children with atopic dermatitis. *Journal of Pediatrics*, **115**, 23–27.

Sampson, H.A., Broadbent, K.R. and Bernhisel-Broadbent, J. (1989) Spontaneous release of histamine from basophils and food hypersensitivity. *New England Journal of Medicine*, **321**, 228–232.

Sandberg, D.H. (1977) Severe steroid response nephrosis associated with food hypersensitivity. *Lancet*, **i**, 388–392.

Uhnoo, I.S., Freihorst, J., Riepenhoff-Talty, M. *et al.* (1990) Effect of rotavirus infection and malnutrition on uptake of a dietary antigen in the intestine. *Pediatric Research*, **27**, 153–160.

Valenta, R., Duchene, M., Ebner, C. *et al.* (1992) Profilins constitute a novel family of functional plant pan-allergens. *Journal of Experimental Medicine*, **175**, 377–385.

Van Asperen, P.P., Kemp, A.S. and Melli, C.M. (1983) Immediate food hypersensitivity reactions on the first known exposure to the food. *Archives of Diseases in Childhood*, **58**, 253–256.

Ventura, A., Longo, G., Longo, F. *et al.* (1989) Diet and atopic eczema in children. *Allergy*, **44**, (Suppl. 9), 159–164.

Walker, W.A. and Isselbacher, K.J. (1974) Uptake and transport of macromolecules by the intestine: possible role in clinical disorders. *Gastroenterology*, **67**, 531–550.

Warner, J.O. (1980) Food allergy in fully breast fed infants. *Clinical Allergy*, **10**, 133–136.

Wüthrich, B. (1983) [Allergic and pseudoallergic reactions of the skin from medicines and food additives.] *Schweizerische Rundschau Med*, **72**, 691–699.

Wüthrich, B. and Hofer, Th. (1986) [Food allergy. III. Treatment: elimination diets, prevention of clinical symptoms and desensitization.] *Schweizerische Med Qschr*, **116**, 1401–1410.

Zeiger, R.S., Heller, S., Mellon, M.H. *et al.* (1989) Effect of combined maternal and infant food allergen avoidance on development of atopy in early infancy: a randomized study. *Journal of Allergy and Clinical Immunology*, **84**, 72–89.

9
Energy density of weaning foods

Alizon Draper

World Cancer Research Fund, 11–12 Buckingham Gate, London SW1E 6LB, UK

INTRODUCTION

Weaning is a period of transition for the infant during which its diet changes in terms of consistency and source: from a liquid milk-based diet the child is gradually introduced to a semi-solid and then a solid diet based on local staples. The young child is very vulnerable at this time and the phrase 'the weanling's dilemma' has been used to refer to the potential risks attendant on weaning. This refers primarily to the risk of contamination of weaning foods with pathogens and the question of when to initiate weaning (Rowland, 1986), but the infant is also vulnerable because of its high nutritional requirements in relation to body size due to the demands of growth. In many developing countries, it has been observed that growth of breast-fed infants is comparable to their counterparts from developed countries until about 3–6 months of age, when breast milk alone is no longer sufficient to meet the needs of the growing infant and supplementary foods need to be introduced. This faltering in growth is attributed to the synergic effects of infection and inadequate dietary intake due to the poor nutritional quality of weaning diets in developing countries, and in particular their low energy density.

There is no standard definition of the term weaning. Rowland's definition of weaning as the 'regular administration of additional food to the breast-fed child' which 'commences with the first of these regular additions and ends with the cessation of breast feeding' (Rowland, 1986)

Infant Nutrition. Edited by A.F. Walker and B.A. Rolls.
Published in 1994 by Chapman & Hall, London.
ISBN 0 412 59140 5.

is used here, with the qualification of Dearden *et al.* (1980) that the completion of weaning also includes the complete transition to the general or adult diet. Weaning practices around the world are very varied with regard to when supplementary foods are introduced into the infant's diet, what foods are given and how long breast feeding is continued. In some countries, weaning foods are given as a supplement to breast milk before 4 months of age, and the length of time breast feeding is continued may vary from under 6 months to over 2 years. In most developing countries, weaning spans a period from about 4 months to about 3 years (Dearden *et al.* 1980). The actual method of infant feeding (i.e. spoon versus hand or bottle feeding) also varies, and this, as discussed later, may have implications for the provision of nutritionally adequate weaning foods. In many developing countries, children are traditionally weaned onto a gruel or porridge made from local staple foods, such as cereals or tubers. These gruels tend to have a low energy density, that is the amount of energy per unit volume of food, of only about 1.3 kJ/g (0.3 kcal/g) compared with a value of 2.9 kJ/g (0.7 kcal/g) for breast milk and a value that can be as high as 5.9 kJ/g (1.4 kcal/g) for a typical UK weaning food (Walker and Pavitt, 1989). This low energy density has been identified as one of the factors in the aetiology of malnutrition in infants and young children (e.g. Rutishauser, 1974; Church, 1979; Dearden *et al.* 1980; Ljungqvist *et al.* 1981; Svanberg, 1987; Walker and Pavitt, 1989; Walker, 1990).

The problem as it has been defined is, in essence, that when the energy density of the weaning food is low, the quantity that must be eaten to satisfy nutritional requirements will be in excess of the amount a small child can actually eat. As previously discussed, low energy density is usually associated with weaning foods made from starchy staples. However, with the rise in popularity of vegetarianism in the West, concern has recently been expressed about the adequacy of vegetarian diets used for weaning, since it has been observed in a number of Western countries that vegetarian children tend to be both shorter and lighter than their omnivorous counterparts (Purves and Sanders, 1980; Dwyer *et al.* 1983; Dagnelie *et al.* 1989). Opinions differ regarding the adequacy of vegetarian diets for young children, but it is the more strict vegetarian diets, such as veganism and macrobiotics, that are likely to have a low energy density (Jacobs and Dwyer, 1988; Nutrition Standing Committee of the British Paediatric Association, 1988). Low energy density is, however, part of the broader problem of dietary bulk.

'Dietary bulk' is a term that is often used somewhat loosely, and it is not always clear whether it is being used to refer to volume or consistency, but Svanberg (1987) describes the term as properly referring to the high volume : viscosity characteristic of a diet. The 'bulk' of a diet is inversely related to its energy density, and a 'bulky' diet will have a low energy

density and viscosity but a high volume. The energy intake of infants and young children will thus be constrained by low energy density if the 'bulk' of their diet is limiting their food intake.

FOOD FACTORS RELATED TO LOW ENERGY DENSITY

The low energy density of traditional weaning foods and some vegetarian diets is a product primarily of their low fat content combined with a high starch content and its particular cooking characteristics. Starch is a polysaccharide composed of long chains of glucose, and it is present in plants as a storage material in the form of granules. There are two types of starch – amylose (straight chain) and amylopectin (branched chain) – and their ratio varies in different starchy foods. The starch content of plant foods also varies, but as a group cereals contain about 40–80% starch dry weight, tubers about 60–80% dry weight, and pulses about 30–40% dry weight. Some fruits, such as plantain, also have a high starch content (about 70%).

When starch is cooked with water the granules start to swell at about 55–70 °C, the initial gelatinization temperature which varies with the type of starch. Continued heating increases the swelling, resulting in a marked increase in viscosity or consistency. The viscosity rises until, at about 85 °C, the starch granules start to collapse and disperse in the water. When the starch chains disperse in the water there is a slight drop in viscosity, but upon cooling the starch sol congeals into a semi-liquid or semi-solid gel. This thick gel has a high water content which is the result of water molecules entering the three-dimensional starch structure (water-holding) and/or water molecules being bound to exposed polar groups on the starch (water-binding). Starches from different food sources behave differently when cooked owing to differences in the size of the starch granules (large granules swell more than small ones), variations in the amylose : amylopectin ratio (amylose swells more than amylopectin), and differences in other food constituents, such as lipids and proteins, which can modify the viscosity potential of starch.

Because of these cooking characteristics, to prepare a gruel or porridge from starchy staple foods with the appropriate liquid or semi-solid consistency for infant feeding requires the addition of large amounts of liquid, usually water. This dilution results in a marked reduction in the concentration of food solids and energy, and a corresponding increase in the volume of the porridge that must be consumed to cover energy requirements.

The low energy density of some Western vegetarian diets is caused by the same factors (that is, a low fat and a high starch content). Given the diversity of vegetarian diets it is hard to generalize, but energy density tends to decrease with increasing avoidance of animal foods. Vegetarian

diets that include dairy products tend to be lower in bulk and pose fewer problems during weaning than more restrictive regimens, such as veganism, macrobiotics or Rastafarianism. These diets often have a low energy density and also shortfalls of other nutrients, such as vitamin D and calcium. The adequacy of different types of vegetarian diet for weaning have been reviewed by Jacobs and Dwyer (1988) and the Nutrition Standing Committee of the British Paediatric Committee (1988).

LOW ENERGY DENSITY AS A LIMITING FACTOR FOR THE ENERGY INTAKE OF YOUNG CHILDREN

Nicol (1971) was one of the first to attempt to quantify the problem of dietary bulk and low energy density by calculating the amounts of different staple foods that children of different age groups would have to consume to cover their energy needs. He estimated that the volume of a cereal-based diet needed to meet the requirements of 1–3-year-old children was 690 ml, which he considered them capable of eating if they were fed frequently enough (four times a day). However, with a diet based on starchy roots like cassava, children in this age group would have to eat 1450 ml of sticky porridge, which he considered an excessive and impossible amount for a young child. Nicol, however, did not include estimations of energy density or measurements of viscosity in his calculations.

Viscosity or consistency is another very important quality of weaning foods, since infants cannot tolerate a solid diet as neither their digestive physiology nor their eating skills are fully developed. With decreasing age and during illness there is an increasing preference for more liquid foods; an infant of about 6 months cannot feed itself and requires foods of a semi-solid or liquid consistency, but a child of about 2 years old can feed itself and is able to eat a solid diet. Church (1979) addressed the problem of the energy density of weaning foods in relation to viscosity and the viscosities appropriate for children of different ages and during illness. He illustrated the inverse relationship between viscosity and energy density that characterizes most traditional weaning foods; to produce a food with a drinkable consistency requires the addition of water to approximately 950 kg water/kg, but at this level of dilution the energy density will only be about 1 kJ/g (0.25 kcal/g). For a 1-year-old child to achieve an energy intake of 1000 kcal (~4.2 MJ), it would have to consume 4 litres of a gruel of this viscosity and energy density, which is obviously not feasible. Mosha and Svanberg (1983) define the viscosity appropriate for young child feeding as 1000–3000 cP (1–3 Pa s) which corresponds to a liquid to semi-liquid consistency. In gruels prepared from cereal flours this is achieved with approximately 10% dry matter and an energy density of about 1.3 kJ/g (0.3 kcal/g).

The food intake necessary to cover the energy needs of children of different ages with diets of different energy densities and viscosities can thus be calculated using published values for energy requirements. However, to define an optimal energy density for weaning foods requires knowledge of the eating capacity of young children. As Ljungqvist *et al.* (1981) note, it should be theoretically possible to calculate this from stomach volume, gastric emptying rate and feeding frequency, but in practice all these factors vary. Hence, estimation of the eating capacity of young children has to be based upon studies of actual dietary intake in infants and young children. However, the accurate and valid measurement of voluntary dietary intake in infants and young children is particularly difficult, since they cannot feed themselves and their intake is influenced by many external factors, such as adult supervision. Unfortunately, there have been few rigorous studies that have attempted to measure the eating capacity of young children, and/or addressed the effect of dietary bulk and energy density in relation to the energy intake of infants and young children.

STUDIES OF FOOD INTAKE IN YOUNG CHILDREN

Rutishauser (1974) investigated the relative influence of several factors on the energy intake of pre-school children. These included feeding frequency, dietary bulk and energy density, 'appetite', infection, seasonality and breast feeding. Dietary intake was estimated using the 24-hour recall method at monthly intervals over a period from 6 months to 3 years. During the first year of life, the principal factors determining energy and protein intakes were the small amounts of food offered to the children in addition to breast milk, and – after 6 months of age – poor appetite, which was often associated with infection. For children over 1 year old, breast feeding made a significant contribution to energy intake, and even those who had good appetites had very low energy intakes if they were no longer breast-fed. Rutishauser concluded that the bulkiness and low energy density of the traditional diet was one of the factors limiting energy intake, particularly since most children were only fed twice a day, and traditional weaning foods were unable to compensate for the cessation of breast feeding.

This finding was confirmed in another study (Rutishauser and Frood, 1973) on the food intake and growth of two groups of Ugandan children aged 1–3 years under supervision in a metabolic ward. The children, all of whom had signs of early clinical malnutrition, were divided into two groups, one of which was fed on a milk-based diet, and the other on a diet based on the food usually consumed at home. All the children were fed five times a day. The total amount of solids and liquids ingested was

similar in both groups, but the energy and protein intakes (both gross and per kilogram body weight) of the group fed on the home diet were significantly lower than those of the children given the milk-based diet. Increase in body weight was also significantly higher in the group given the milk-based diet. Even when fed five times daily, which is more frequent than the customary two or three times reported by the mothers, the children given the home diet had difficulty covering their energy needs. With regard to dietary bulk, the authors concluded that a mean daily intake of over 700 g solid food should be regarded as large and near the maximum eating capacity of children aged 1–3 years.

Other studies on the food intake of infants and young children have found a correlation between energy intake and energy density, confirming that the low energy density of weaning diets is a factor limiting energy intake (Van Steenbergen *et al.* 1980; Araya *et al.* 1983, 1988; Susheela and Rao, 1983). Araya *et al.* (1983) also found that children appeared to be able to modulate their food intake to maintain a constant level of energy intake, but that this only occurred when meals of high energy density were offered. When foods of a low energy density were offered, the children did not increase their food consumption since it appeared to be near maximum gastric capacity. The mean intake of food with the lowest energy density (2 kJ/g; 0.47 kcal/g) at one meal was 495 g.

In a review of studies investigating the food intake of pre-school children, Svanberg (1987) concluded that their maximum eating capacity appears to be about 900–1400 g/day. To satisfy the daily energy requirements of an average healthy 12-month-old child (4.2 MJ, 1000 kcal), the energy density of the diet at the lower level of intake (900 g) would have to meet or exceed 5 kJ/g (1.2 kcal/g), although 2.9 kJ/g (0.7 kcal/g) would be adequate at the upper level of intake. There is even less information regarding the eating capacity of infants. Studies on the intake of milk formula have shown daily intakes ranging from 582 to 899 ml/day in infants under 3 months old (Fomon *et al.* 1969) but, as Svanberg (1987) notes, the relevance of these studies to starch-rich weaning foods is not clear. While the infant is still breast-fed, Svanberg (1987) considers that supplementary weaning foods should have an energy density equivalent to, or exceeding, the energy density of breast milk (2.9 kJ/g; 0.7 kcal/g).

OTHER FACTORS INFLUENCING ENERGY INTAKE

The definition of a desirable energy density of weaning foods is also dependent upon the frequency of feeding, and studies in India have found that increasing the frequency of feeding to four times a day can be effective in enabling children to consume adequate quantities of bulky cereal-based diets (Rau *et al.* 1970; Pasricha, 1973). Increasing the number of

daily feeds can help to increase the food intake of young children, and could be a determining factor in identifying an appropriate energy density for weaning foods between the two extreme values mentioned above (2.9–5.0 kJ/g; 0.7–1.2 kcal/g). However, if the energy density is very low even increasing the feeding frequency to five times a day may not enable a child to consume an adequate quantity of the diet, as Rutishauser and Frood (1973) found. Moreover, increasing the frequency of feeding may not be feasible because the mother or carer may not have enough time, and it is unlikely that feeding frequency with cooked weaning foods could realistically be increased beyond four times a day. Susheela and Rao (1983) consider that, given the customary feeding patterns of two meals a day for rural Indian children, the energy density of the diet should be about 4.2–5.0 kJ/g (1.0–1.2 kcal/g) to ensure an adequate energy intake.

The definition of an optimal energy density for weaning foods is thus dependent upon related factors, such as frequency of feeding and the eating capacity of infants and young children, all of which vary. More research is needed to identify the optimal energy density of weaning foods, and also to investigate the effect of viscosity on the volume of food consumed by young children, which has not been addressed. The difficulty of defining an appropriate energy density is further confounded by the continuing uncertainty regarding the energy requirements of infants and young children (Walker, 1990). It also needs to be remembered that the food intake of infants and young children is affected by a range of wider influences, such as the quality of adult supervision. In a study on the value of the traditional Ghanaian diet in relation to the energy needs of young children (1–3 years), Woolfe *et al.* (1977) found that the traditional diet and pattern of feeding could satisfy the energy needs of the children studied, but that a wide range of food intakes was observed. This was attributed to the quantity of food offered to children and, more importantly, the amount of encouragement to eat that the children received (Figure 9.1).

Another factor that has received little attention is the actual method of child feeding. For instance, bottle feeding is very common in many parts of the world. It is less demanding upon the mother or carer since the child can feed itself, but it requires that the weaning food be of a liquid consistency. This inevitably results in diluted gruels of low energy density being given to the child. In a study of infant feeding practices in Nigeria, Oni *et al.* (1990) found that hand feeding infants was common in both rural and urban areas. Hand feeding, like bottle feeding, requires that the foods offered are liquid or semi-liquid. Mothers also believed that younger children were not developmentally ready for solid foods. The authors suggest, however, that hand feeding may be culturally adaptive, since the locally available staple foods yield viscous foods when the amount of food

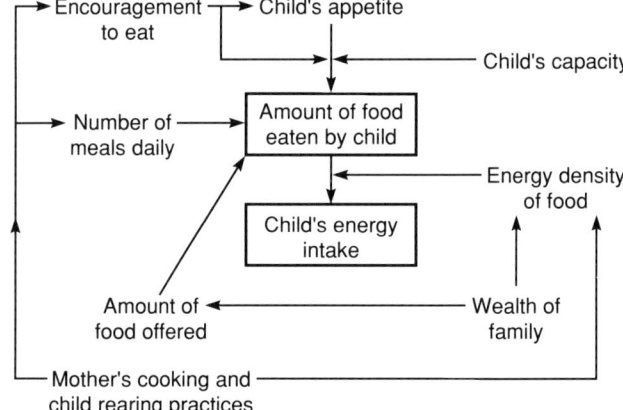

Figure 9.1 Some of the factors affecting the food and energy intake of a young child. (From Woolfe *et al.* 1977.)

solids exceed 8–10%, and hand feeding may be the only way to encourage the child to consume the necessary volume of the dilute feeds to cover energy requirements, particularly if a child is ill. Hand feeding is also a very time-efficient method of child feeding – an important consideration for women burdened with domestic work and economic activities. In conclusion, the authors point to the need for further research into the potential advantages of hand feeding in relation to the other factors that influence children's nutrition and women's available time.

There is a wide range of factors other than low energy density, such as frequency and method of feeding, that influence the energy intake of young children. Pelto (1984) has outlined the range of sociocultural factors that may influence infant feeding and nutrition. Despite the difficulty of defining an appropriate energy density for weaning foods and the need for further research in this area, increasing the energy density of weaning foods may be the most feasible intervention to increase the energy intake of infants and young children in developing countries. Ways to increase it are now discussed.

WAYS OF INCREASING THE ENERGY DENSITY OF WEANING FOODS

There are essentially two ways of reducing the dietary bulk of weaning foods and increasing energy density: through the addition of energy-rich supplements such as oils or fats, and through modification of the starch content of weaning foods. Both are effective, but there are many factors that may compromise the efficacy and acceptability of these methods in practice. These constraints are largely dependent upon the particular socioeconomic and cultural context of child feeding. Recently there has been much interest in the potential of traditional technologies, particularly germination and fermentation, to improve the feeding of young children (see Alnwick *et al.* 1988). Because these technologies are already used in many parts of the world, they would appear to be more appropriate and culturally acceptable and hence more effective and sustainable methods of increasing the energy density of weaning diets. Unfortunately, despite the proven efficacy of some of these methods in laboratory studies, there have been few community trials to assess their acceptability and efficacy in reducing malnutrition in young children. These technologies also carry a risk of undesirable side effects, such as contamination with mycotoxins or the production of cyanide.

Addition of energy

This is the simplest and most straightforward way to increase energy density through the addition of an energy-rich supplement, such as sugar or fat. Since fats and oils are the most energy-dense food components (they provide 37 kJ/g (9 kcal/g) compared with 16–17 kJ/g (4 kcal/g) from carbohydrate or protein) they are usually suggested as the most effective (Srikantia, 1979; Dearden *et al.* 1980). Some fats have an effect upon the viscosity of starch pastes, although the effects vary and depend upon the type of fat used (Walker and Pavitt, 1989). Fat also increases the palatability of food, although Dearden *et al.* (1980) warn against the addition of an excessive amount of fat because its high satiety value could lead to a reduced food intake and could also have a detrimental affect upon protein intake (Walker, 1990). An alternative is the addition of a supplement rich in both energy and protein, such as peanut butter, provided it is free from aflatoxin. Potential constraints on the use of energy-rich supplements are cost and availability and attitudes regarding their suitability for young children.

Modification of starch content

The swelling properties of starch may be modified in various ways to prevent it forming thick viscous porridges when cooked which require dilution. This may be done by physical means, such as extrusion or flaking, or by chemical means, such as germination. These may be either traditional or more modern methods of food processing.

Extrusion is a modern food-processing technique which is used in many countries to produce weaning foods. It carries various advantages and disadvantages. The technique is versatile and allows a wide variety of locally available ingredients to be used, and the product can be fortified with additional vitamins or flavourings if desired. The resultant product is ready to eat, and can easily be mixed with milk or water. Moreover, because of damage to the starch molecules during processing, gruels made from extruded ingredients have been reported to have higher energy densities than non-extruded gruels (Jansen *et al.* 1981). The heat treatment also removes some anti-nutritional factors, but reduces the nutritional quality of some proteins, for instance by reducing available lysine. Despite the development of low-cost extrusion cookers (Jansen and Harper, 1980a, 1980b), they remain expensive pieces of equipment which require skilled personnel to run them.

There are several traditional technologies practised at the household level which have recently been identified as having a potential to increase the energy density of weaning diets and so improve young child feeding. Of these, germination, and more specifically the use of amylase-rich foods (ARF) produced by germination, would appear to hold the most potential.

Germination or malting is the sprouting of cereal and legume grains which is brought about by soaking the grain in water. This stimulates metabolic activity as the seed starts to grow. A number of complex changes occur during this process, such as the breakdown of storage materials, including starch, and the synthesis of new substances, such as vitamins. These changes alter the flavour, cooking properties, shelf life and nutritional qualities of foods made from germinated grains. Of pertinence here is the synthesis of amylase enzymes, which digest starch and break it down into dextrins and maltose. Because the products of starch hydrolysis do not gelatinize when cooked, the germination of grains can have a marked effect upon the viscosity of starch porridges.

The germination of grains has been shown to have a dramatic effect upon the viscosity and energy density of porridges made from fully malted cereal flours and combinations of malted cereals and legumes (Desikachar, 1980; Brandtzaeg *et al.* 1981; Gopaldas *et al.* 1982; Mosha and Svanberg, 1983; Marero *et al.* 1988a, 1988b). A porridge of appropriate consistency can be prepared using malted flours at concentrations up to 25% (the concentration varying with cereal variety), which compares with about 10% for porridges made from unmalted flours. More recently, however, the efficacy of adding a small amount of malted flour to cooked porridge in order to liquefy it has been explored (Gopaldas *et al.* 1986, 1988; Atwell *et al.* 1988; John and Gopaldas, 1988; Hansen *et al.* 1989). These malts have been referred to as ARF and have been shown to be very effective in reducing the viscosity of thick porridges. The energy density of a porridge thinned with an ARF varies, but in general the dry matter content and hence energy density can be increased by two or three times.

In practice, however, the efficacy of germination and ARF is compromised by several factors: the amylolytic activity of different varieties of grain varies considerably, and also depends upon the physical conditions of germination; the cooking procedure used to prepare weaning foods can affect the ability of ARF to reduce viscosity and so increase energy density; some malted grains have a limited shelf life, although this is also dependent upon post-germination processing. The germination of grains may carry certain undesirable side effects, such as contamination with aflatoxin-producing moulds and diarrhoeal pathogens during storage and, when sorghum grains are used, the production of cyanide. Although it has been clearly established that both fully malted flours and ARF can reduce the viscosity and increase the energy density of starchy porridges, the results of feeding trials are ambiguous and do not clearly indicate the effectiveness of germination in improving infant and child feeding. There has been little experience or evaluation of their promotion and there is a need for further research, particularly at the community level. The cultural acceptability of germination in relation to child feeding, and the costs involved in terms of utensils, time, labour and space also need attention.

Parching, puffing, roasting and flaking are traditional Indian food technologies which are used to process cereal and legume grains at the household level. They have attracted some attention because of their ability to modify the viscosity of weaning foods (Desikachar, 1980, 1982; Gopaldas *et al.* 1986). The more severe treatments, such as puffing and flaking, have been found to reduce the viscosity of gruels but the effect is not as great as that produced by germinating grains.

Fermentation is one of the oldest techniques of food processing practised by humankind, and is the result of the activity of microorganisms (yeasts, moulds or bacteria) as they utilize the organic components of food to obtain energy for growth. It is essentially a catabolic process in which complex molecules are broken down and utilized for energy. There are an enormous number of different fermentation processes which vary according to the type and composition of the fermentation substrate, the

Table 9.1 The relationship between consistency, dietary bulk and energy density in maize porridge

Consistency	Percentage solids	Energy density (kJ/ml)	(kcal/ml)	Volume that provides 4.2 MJ or 1000 kcal[a] (ml)
Thin	10	1.5	0.36	2778
Semi-solid	15	2.3	0.54	1842
Stiff	20	3.0	0.72	1390

[a]The daily energy requirement of an average healthy child aged 12 months.

microorganisms present and the conditions of fermentation such as pH and temperature. The microbiology of fermented porridges, which are popular in many parts of Africa, has recently attracted attention. Despite many allusions in the literature to the viscosity-reducing effects of fermentation (e.g. Lechtig and Srivastava, 1988; Nout *et al.* 1988), this is rarely substantiated, and there has been little work specifically addressing the effect of fermentation on viscosity and energy density. The findings of the work that has been carried out are highly contradictory, and appear to depend on the method of fermentation and in particular the microorganisms involved. Steinkraus (1990, personal communication) considers that the lactic acid bacterial fermentations, which are involved in the preparation of sour cereal- and tuber-based porridges, will have little effect since there are few, if any, amylolytic enzymes present to digest the starch. Microorganisms involved in other fermentation processes have been found to produce amylase enzymes (Akinrele, 1970), but their ability to digest starch may be inhibited by the low pH of fermented foods. The potential of fermentation to increase the energy density of weaning foods is thus an area requiring further research.

The fermentation of foodstuffs, however, confers other well documented nutritional benefits and generally results in increased flavour, digestibility and nutritive value. Fermented foods have enhanced organoleptic properties which are valuable when a child's appetite may be reduced, for instance during illness, and there has been some interest in their potential for use as a food-based oral rehydration therapy. It has also been shown that fermentation reduces the contamination and proliferation of diarrhoeal pathogens (Mensah *et al.* 1988, 1990), although the actual mechanism by which this occurs is not yet known. Further research is needed in these areas and to ensure that there are no contraindications to the use of fermented foods for weaning.

CONCLUSIONS

The low energy density of weaning foods is often referred to as limiting the energy intake of infants and young children in developing countries. However, this claim is based upon only a small number of studies. There is need for further research to investigate the precise effects of dietary bulk, energy density and viscosity on the energy intake of infants and young children. The adequacy of a particular weaning food with regard to energy density also needs to be seen in the context of specific local patterns of infant feeding, such as the method and frequency of feeding. In the light of present knowledge it is therefore not possible to define a single precise value for the optimal energy density of weaning foods, although it would appear that a value of about 2.9 kJ/g (0.7 kcal/g) represents a lower limit. Various ways, both traditional and non-traditional, in which the energy density of weaning foods can be increased have been discussed, but again there is still need for further work to develop feasible and acceptable methods.

REFERENCES

Akinrele, I.A. (1970) Fermentation studies on maize during the preparation of a traditional African starch-cake food. *Journal of the Science of Food and Agriculture*, **21**, 619–625.

Alnwick, D., Moses, S. and Schmidt, O. G. (1988) *Improving Young Child Feeding in Eastern and Southern Africa: Household-Level Food Technology*. Ottawa: IDRC.

Araya, H., Vera, G. and Pak, N. (1983) Effect of dietary energy density on food intake of preschool children in one meal. *Nutrition Reports International*, **28**, 965–971.

Araya, H., Vera, G. and Pak, N. (1988) An experimental model to establish recommended values of energy density of diets for preschool children. *Nutrition Reports International*, **37**, 241–248.

Atwell, W.A., Hyldon, R.G., Godfrey, P.D. *et al.* (1988) Germinated quinoa flour to reduce the viscosity of starchy foods. *Cereal Chemistry*, **65**, 508–509.

Brandtzaeg, B., Malleshi, N.G., Svanberg, U. *et al.* (1981) Dietary bulk as a limiting factor for nutrient intake – with special reference to the feeding of pre-school children. III. Studies of malted flour from ragi, sorghum and green gram. *Journal of Tropical Pediatrics*, **27**, 184–189.

Church, M. (1979) Dietary factors in malnutrition: quality and quantity of diet in relation to child development. *Proceedings of the Nutrition Society*, **38**, 41–49.

Dagnelie, P.C., van Staveren, W.A., Vergote, F.J.V.R.A. *et al.* (1989) Nutritional status of infants aged 4 to 18 months on macrobiotic diets and matched omnivorous controls: a population-based mixed-longitudinal study. II. Growth and psychomotor development. *European Journal of Clinical Nutrition*, **43**, 325–338.

Dearden, C., Harman, P. and Morley, D. (1980) Eating more fats and oils as a step towards overcoming malnutrition. *Tropical Doctor*, **10**, 137–142.

Desikachar, H.S.R. (1980) Development of weaning foods with high caloric density and low hot-paste viscosity using traditional technologies. *Food and Nutrition Bulletin*, **2**, 21–23.

Desikachar, H.S.R. (1982) Technology options for formulating weaning foods for the economically weaker segments of populations in developing countries. *Food and Nutrition Bulletin*, **4**, 57–59.

Dwyer, J.T., Andrew, E.M., Berkey, C. *et al.* (1983) Growth in 'new' vegetarian preschool children using the Jenss–Bayley curve fitting technique. *American Journal of Clinical Nutrition*, **37**, 815–827.

Fomon, S.J., Filer, L.J., Thomas, L.N. *et al.* (1969) Relationship between formula concentration and rate of growth of normal infants. *Journal of Nutrition*, **98**, 241–254.

Gopaldas, T., Despande, S. and John, C. (1988) Studies on a wheat-based amylase-rich food. *Food and Nutrition Bulletin*, **10**, 55–59.

Gopaldas, T., Inamdar, F. and Patel, J. (1982) Malted versus roasted young child mixes: viscosity, storage and acceptability trials. *Indian Journal of Nutrition and Dietetics*, **19**, 327–336.

Gopaldas, T., Mehta, P., Patil, A. and Ghandi, H. (1986) Studies on reduction in viscosity of thick rice gruels with small quantities of an amylase-rich cereal malt. *Food and Nutrition Bulletin*, **8**, 42–47.

Hansen, M., Pedersen, B., Munck, L. and Eggum, B.O. (1989) Weaning foods with improved energy and nutrient density prepared from germinated cereals. I. Preparation and dietary bulk of gruels based on barley. *Food and Nutrition Bulletin*, **11**, 40–45.

Jacobs, C. and Dwyer, J.T. (1988) Vegetarian children: appropriate and inappropriate diets. *American Journal of Clinical Nutrition*, **48**, 811–818.

Jansen, G.R. and Harper, J.M. (1980a) Application of low-cost extrusion cooking to weaning foods in feeding programmes. Part 1. *Food and Nutrition*, **6**, 2–9.

Jansen, G.R. and Harper, J.M. (1980b) Application of low-cost extrusion cooking to weaning foods in feeding programmes. Part 2. *Food and Nutrition*, **6**, 15–23.

Jansen, G.R., O'Deen, L., Tribelhorn, R.E. and Harper, J.M. (1981) The calorie densities of gruels made from extruded corn–soy blends. *Food and Nutrition Bulletin*, **3**, 39–44.

John, C. and Gopaldas, T. (1988) Reduction in the dietary bulk of soya-fortified bulghur wheat gruels with wheat-based amylase-rich food. *Food and Nutrition Bulletin*, **10**, 50–53.

Lechtig, A. and Srivastava, S. (1988) A strategy to improve weaning practices in Mozambique. In *Improving Young Child Feeding in Eastern and Southern Africa: Household-Level Food Technology*, pp. 113–127 (eds D. Alnwick, S. Moses and O.G. Schmidt). Ottawa: IDRC.

Ljungqvist, B., Mellander, O. and Svanberg, U. (1981) Dietary bulk as a limiting factor for nutrient intake in pre-school children. I. A problem description. *Journal of Tropical Pediatrics*, **27**, 68–73.

Marero, L.M., Payumo, E.M., Aguinaldo, A.R. and Homma, S. (1988a) Nutritional characteristics of weaning foods prepared from germinated cereals and legumes. *Journal of Food Science*, **53**, 1399–1402.

Marero, L.M., Payumo, E.M., Librando, E.C. *et al.* (1988b) Technology of weaning food formulations prepared from germinated cereals and legumes. *Journal of Food Science*, **53**, 1391–1395.

Mensah, P., Tomkins, A., Drasar, B.S. and Harrison, T.J. (1988) Effect of fermentation of Ghanaian maize dough on the survival and proliferation of 4 strains of Shigella flexneri. *Transactions of the Royal Society of Tropical Medicine and Hygiene*, **82**, 635–636.

Mensah, P., Tomkins, A., Drasar, B.S. and Harrison, T.J. (1990) Fermentation of cereals for reduction of bacterial contamination of weaning foods in Ghana. *Lancet*, **336**, 140–143.

Mosha, A.C. and Svanberg, U. (1983) Preparation of weaning foods with high nutrient density using flour of germinated cereals. *Food and Nutrition Bulletin*, **5**, 10–14.

Nicol, B.M. (1971) Protein and calorie concentration. *Nutrition Reviews*, **29**, 83–88.

Nout, M.J.R., Hautvast, J.G.A.J., van der Haar, F. *et al.* (1988) Formulation and microbiological safety of cereal-based weaning foods. In *Improving Young Child Feeding in Eastern and Southern Africa: Household-Level Food Technology*, pp. 245–260 (eds D. Alnwick, S. Moses and O.G. Schmidt). Ottawa: IDRC.

Nutrition Standing Committee of the British Paediatric Association (1988) Vegetarian weaning. *Archives of Disease in Childhood*, **63**, 1286–1292.

Oni, G.A., Brown, K.H., Bentley, M.E. *et al.* (1990) Feeding practices and prevalence of hand-feeding of infants and young children in Kwara State, Nigeria. *Ecology of Food and Nutrition*, 25, 1–11.

Pasricha, S. (1973) Possible calorie intakes in young children fed cereal based diets. *Indian Journal of Nutrition and Dietetics*, 10, 282–285.

Pelto, G.H. (1984) Ethnographic studies of the effects of food availability and infant feeding practices. *Food and Nutrition Bulletin*, 6, 33–43.

Purves, R. and Sanders, T.A.B. (1980) An assessment of the nutritional status of preschool vegan children. *Proceedings of the Nutrition Society*, 39, 79A.

Rau, M.P., Rao, D.H., Naidu, A.N. and Swaminathan, M.C. (1970) Calorie intake of pre-school children when fed *ad lib*. *Indian Journal of Nutrition and Dietetics*, 7, 337–341.

Rowland, M.G.M. (1986) The weanling's dilemma: are we making progress? *Acta Paediatrica Scandinavica*, 323, 33–42.

Rutishauser, I.H.E. (1974) Factors affecting the intake of energy and protein by Ugandan preschool children. *Ecology of Food and Nutrition*, 3, 213–222.

Rutishauser, I.H.E. and Frood, J.D.L. (1973) The effect of a traditional low-fat diet on energy and protein intake, serum albumin concentration and bodyweight in Ugandan preschool children. *British Journal of Nutrition*, 29, 261–268.

Srikantia, S.G. (1979) Use of fats and oils in child feeding. *Food and Nutrition*, 5, 18–22.

Susheela, T.P. and Rao, B.S.N. (1983) Energy density of diet in relation to energy intake of preschool children from urban and rural communities of different economic status. *Human Nutrition: Clinical Nutrition*, 37C, 133–137.

Svanberg, U. (1987) *Dietary Bulk in Weaning Foods*. Göteborg, Sweden: Department of Food Science, Chalmers University of Technology.

Van Steenbergen, W.M., Kusin, J.A. and Jansen, A.A.J. (1980) Measured food intake of preschool children in Machakos district. *East African Medical Journal*, 57, 734–744.

Walker, A.F. (1990) The contribution of weaning foods to protein-energy malnutrition. *Nutrition Research Reviews*, 3, 25–47.

Walker, A.F. and Pavitt, F. (1989) Energy density of Third World weaning foods. *BNF Nutrition Bulletin*, 14, 88–101.

Woolfe, J.A., Wheeler, E.G., van Dyke, W. and Orraca-Tetteh, R. (1977) The value of the Ghanaian traditional diet in relation to the energy needs of young children. *Ecology of Food and Nutrition*, 6, 175–181.

Index

Page numbers in **bold** represent figures and those in *italics* represent tables.